The Thirty-ninth Hahnemann
Endocrinology-Metabolism Symposium

New Concepts in
Endocrinology and Metabolism

The Thirty-ninth Hahnemann
Endocrinology-Metabolism Symposium

New Concepts in Endocrinology and Metabolism

Editors

Leslie I. Rose, M.D.

*Associate Professor of Medicine
and Director, Division of Endocrinology and Metabolism
Hahnemann Medical College and Hospital
Philadelphia, Pennsylvania*

Robert L. Lavine, M.D.

*Assistant Professor of Medicine
Division of Endocrinology and Metabolism
and Director, Diabetic Clinics
Hahnemann Medical College and Hospital
Philadelphia, Pennsylvania*

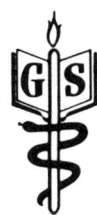

GRUNE & STRATTON
A Subsidiary of Harcourt Brace Jovanovich, Publishers
New York   San Francisco   London

Library of Congress Cataloging in Publication Data

Hahnemann Endocrinology–Metabolism Symposium, Philadelphia, 1976.
  New concepts in endocrinology and metabolism.

  Includes bibliographical references and index.
  1. Endocrine glands—Diseases—Congresses.
2. Diabetes—Congresses. 3. Metabolism, Disorders of—Congresses. I. Rose, Leslie I. II. Lavine, Robert L. III. Hahnemann Medical College and Hospital of Philadelphia. IV. Title. [DNLM:
1. Endocrinology—Congresses. WK100 N532 1976]
RC648.A1H33 1976   616.4   77-9314
ISBN 0-8089-1027-2

© *1977 by Grune & Stratton, Inc.*
All rights reserved. No part of this publication may be reproduced or transmitted in any form or by any means, electronic or mechanical, including photocopy, recording, or any information storage and retrieval system, without permission in writing from the publisher.

Grune & Stratton, Inc.
111 Fifth Avenue
New York, New York 10003

Distributed in the United Kindom by
Academic Press, Inc. (London) Ltd.
24/48 Oval Road, London NW 1

Library of Congress Catalog Number 77-9314
International Standard Book Number 0-8089-1027-2
Printed in the United States of America

Contents

Preface   vii

Contributors   viii

1. Physiologic Precepts for Evaluation of Thyroid Function Tests   1
   Herbert A. Selenkow

2. Diagnosis and Treatment of Hypothyroidism   19
   Robert D. Utiger

3. T3 Toxicosis and Its Clinical Variants: A Reappraisal   37
   Stephen Richardson and Charles S. Hollander

4. Diagnosis and Treatment of Adrenocortical Insufficiency   49
   Robert G. Dluhy

5. Diagnosis and Treatment of Cushing's Syndrome   57
   David H. P. Streeten, Theodore G. Dalakos, and Gunnar H. Anderson, Jr.

6. Renin-Angiotensin-Aldosterone Axis and Hypertension   73
   Gordon H. Williams

7. An Approach to the Hypertensive Patient   83
   Paul G. Cohen

8. Evaluation and Therapy of the Hirsute Female   87
   Leslie I. Rose

9. Medical Management of Renal Calculi   97
   Charles Y. C. Pak, Donald Barilla, Henry Bone, and Cheryl Northcutt

10. Implications from Oral Glucose Tolerance Testing   107
    J. Stuart Soeldner and B. N. Park

11.	The Prudent Physician *Thaddeus E. Prout*	125
12.	Pathophysiology and Treatment of Diabetic Ketoacidosis *Philip Felig*	129
13.	Diabetes and Pregnancy *Robert L. Lavine*	137
14.	Current Treatment of Diabetic Retinopathy *Frank L. Myers*	147
15.	Hyperlipoproteinemia: A Return to the Basics *Peter N. Herbert*	153
	Index	167

Preface

This volume tabulates the results of the Hahnemann Endocrinology-Metabolism Symposium held in February, 1976. It is a compilation of the various presentations given at the symposium and is directed primarily to the practicing physician.

This book does not cover all of the topics that exist in the fields of endocrinology and metabolism, but the chapters concentrate on commonly encountered clinical problems. The authors were chosen because of their expertise in a particular discipline as well as their ability to present their topic in a clear, concise manner. Each author was encouraged to introduce his own bias into his chapter in order to provide guidance to the clinician.

We wish to thank Mr. Robert J. Schaefer, Ms. Jane Krumrine, and Catherine Garofano, R.N., for their help in the organization and conduction of the symposium.

Leslie I. Rose
Robert L. Lavine

Contributors

GUNNAR H. ANDERSON, JR., M.D., Instructor in Medicine, State University of New York Upstate Medical Center, Syracuse, New York

DONALD BARILLA, M.D., Instructor in Internal Medicine, University of Texas Health Science Center, Southwestern Medical School, Dallas, Texas

HENRY BONE, M.D., Instructor in Internal Medicine, University of Texas Health Science Center, Southwestern Medical School, Dallas, Texas

PAUL G. COHEN, M.D., Medical Director, Northside Dialysis Center, Atlanta, Georgia

THEODORE G. DALAKOS, M.D., Assistant Professor of Medicine, State University of New York Upstate Medical Center, Syracuse, New York

ROBERT G. DLUHY, M.D., Associate Professor of Medicine, Harvard Medical School, Boston, Massachusetts

PHILIP FELIG, M.D., Professor and Vice Chairman, Department of Medicine, and Chief, Section of Endocrinology, Yale University School of Medicine, New Haven, Connecticut

PETER N. HERBERT, M.D., Head, Section on Lipoprotein Structure, Molecular Disease Branch, National Heart and Lung Institute, National Institute of Health, Bethesda, Maryland

CHARLES S. HOLLANDER, M.D., Professor of Medicine and Chief, Endocrine Division, and Director, Clinical Research Center, New York University Medical Center, New York, New York

FRANK L. MYERS, M.D., Assistant Clinical Professor, Department of Ophthalmology, University of Wisconsin Medical School, Madison, Wisconsin

CHERYL NORTHCUTT, R.N., Assistant in the Department of Internal Medicine, University of Texas Health Science Center, Southwestern Medical School, Dallas, Texas

CHARLES Y. C. PAK, M.D., Professor of Medicine, University of Texas Health Science Center, Southwestern Medical School, Dallas, Texas

Contributors

B. N. PARK, M.D., formerly Elliott P. Joslin Research Laboratory, Department of Medicine, Peter Bent Brigham Hospital, Harvard Medical School, Boston, Massachusetts

THADDEUS E. PROUT, M.D., Associate Professor of Medicine, Johns Hopkins University School of Medicine, and Chief of Medicine, Greater Baltimore Medical Center, Baltimore, Maryland

STEPHEN RICHARDSON, M.B., M.R.C.P., Researcher in the Endocrine Division, Department of Medicine, New York University School of Medicine, New York, New York

HERBERT A. SELENKOW, M.D., Associate Professor of Medicine, Harvard Medical School, and Endocrine Units, Peter Bent Brigham Hospital, Boston, Massachusetts, and Waltham Hospital, Waltham, Massachusetts

J. STUART SOELDNER, M.D., Associate Professor of Medicine, Harvard Medical School, Boston, Massachusetts

DAVID H. P. STREETEN, M.B., D.Phil., F.R.C.P., Professor of Medicine and Head, Section of Endocrinology, State University of New York Upstate Medical Center, Syracuse, New York

ROBERT D. UTIGER, M.D., Chief, Endocrine Section, Department of Medicine, University of Pennsylvania School of Medicine, Philadelphia, Pennsylvania

GORDON H. WILLIAMS, M.D., Associate Professor of Medicine, Harvard Medical School, Boston, Massachusetts

Herbert A. Selenkow

1
Physiologic Precepts for Evaluation of Thyroid Function Tests

The practicing physician today is confronted with an overwhelming abundance of highly sophisticated and recently developed laboratory aids to diagnosis and therapy. Many of these aids are the results of technologic innovations that are unfamiliar to any but the most recently trained scientists, and the accuracy and diagnostic utility of many of these aids are not yet fully proved. Among these, the recently developed tests of thyroid function appear to partake of this technologic future-shock, for they are marketed in abundant forms and have unstandardized designations or abbreviations and, at times, dissimilar normal ranges and limits of precision. Fortunately, when interpretation of these thyroid function tests is based on sound clinical and physiologic principles, they are remarkably useful; they are rapidly becoming necessary requisites to clinical diagnosis and management.

It is intended in this brief review to present an integrated summary of current physiologic concepts relating to regulation of thyroid hormone synthesis, secretion, and metabolism in order to permit the interested physician to appreciate their clinical application and interpretation. In this regard, several inclusive reviews of this subject are of interest.[1-5]

It is useful to view the regulatory system that controls the secretions and circulating levels of thyroid hormones as an entity with three major interdependent components:

1. The hypothalamic/pituitary/thyroid gland axis
2. The circulating thyroid hormone transport compartment
3. The thyroid hormone tissue metabolism system

Consideration of each of these subsystems individually is useful in understanding the application of specific thyroid function tests to ascertain the physiologic integrity or pathologic alteration of each component. It is now possible to utilize available thyroid function tests with discrimination to localize anatomic sites of thyroidal dysfunction and to monitor responses to clinical therapy.

REGULATION OF THYROID HORMONE SECRETIONS

Hypothalamic/Pituitary/Thyroid Interactions

Secretory regulation of the thyroid gland results in large measure from thyrotropin (TSH) stimulation, which in turn is modulated by two major factors: the serum thyroid hormone concentrations and the availability of the hypothalamic thyrotropin releasing hormone (TRH). These relationships are characterized in simplistic form in Figure 1–1. The metabolic equivalences of both serum free thyroxine (FT4) and free triiodothyronine (FT3) reflect the status of tissue thyrothermic activity and are the most useful current laboratory indicators of thyroid metabolic status. When the combined calorigenic equivalences of serum FT4 and FT3 indicate euthyroidism (regardless of serum ratio of FT4 to FT3), pituitary TSH secretion is retarded to a low point just sufficient to permit a daily thryoid gland secretion of T4 and T3 to maintain euthyroidism. If the serum FT4 and FT3 levels decrease, this signals the hypothalamic release of TRH and a consequent secretion of TSH to stimulate further secretion of hormones until reequilibration of serum levels and tissue levels is achieved. Conversely, if excessive serum and tissue receptor levels of FT4 and FT3 occur, then pituitary TSH is inhibited until the excess hormone is metabolized. The TSH/thyroid axis is regulated by a negative-feedback loop. The TRH/TSH "short" loop may be activated by a positive-feedback mechanism that permits synthesis of TRH during periods of excess thyroid hormone levels and TRH release in response to diminished serum thyroid hormone levels. Persistent excess of serum FT4 and FT3 may produce a state of hypothalamic TRH/TSH inertia, such that administration of exogenous TRH fails to reproduce an adequate TSH response.[6,7] This hypothalamic refractoriness may be utilized to diagnose early or cryptic forms of thyrotoxicosis in a manner similar to use of the thyroid suppression test.

The major characteristics of the hypothalamic/pituitary TRH/TSH short-loop activity are summarized as follows:

1. TRH administration to normal euthyroid subjects produces a characteristic serum TSH pattern with maximal serum concentrations occurring at about 30 min.
2. Release of TSH by TRH in hypothyroid patients is more brisk than normal and results in higher peak serum TSH concentrations.
3. In thyrotoxicosis the TSH response to TRH is blunted or absent. A similar refractoriness occurs in patients who are taking exogenous thyroid hormones, and it persists for 1–2 weeks after discontinuation of thyroid hormones.

Serum TSH concentrations are now readily measurable with excellent precision by use of radioimmunoassay techniques.[8] The serum TSH response to maximal TRH stimulation is measured in microunits per milliliter and is generally in the range of 10–30 μU/ml at peak times. TRH induces a small and transiently measurable rise in serum T3 and a lesser rise in serum T4 that follow the TSH serum peak by 1–4 hr. TRH also stimulates release of pituitary prolactin (HPr) but not other tropic hormones. It is not clear at this time whether (or by what mechanism) serum thyroid hormone concentrations modify TRH secretion or action. The TSH response to TRH in women is slightly greater than in men, and it can be blunted by pharmacologic doses of glucocorticoids, by somatostatin (a growth-hormone-inhibiting peptide), by L-dopa (in therapy of parkinsonism), and by exogenous thyroid hormones.

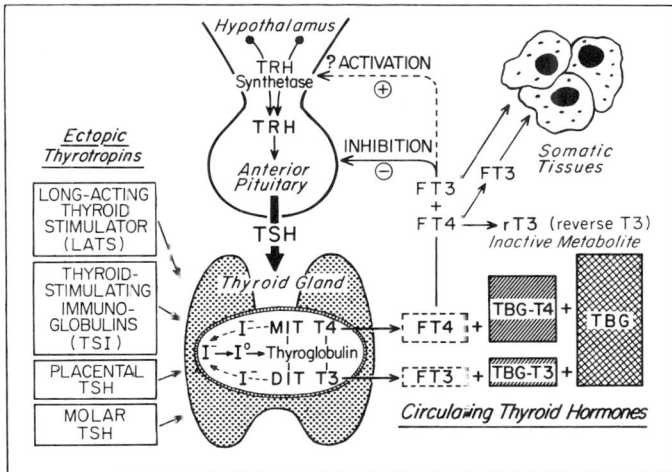

Fig. 1-1. Schematic representation of current concepts of regulation of thyroid hormone secretion. See text for explanation.

Secretion of TSH from the anterior pituitary normally maintains serum levels of this hormone in the range of 1–5 μU/ml as measured by currently available radioimmunoassay methods. When serum levels of free T4 and T3 decline below normal, the hypothalamic/pituitary TRH/TSH response is rapid and persists until euthyroidism is restored in the intact individual. If this is not possible because of thyroid gland failure from whatever reason, serum TSH levels remain persistently elevated. The magnitude of the serum TSH increase varies inversely with the serum FT4 and FT4/FT3 concentrations: the lower the serum FT4/FT3 the greater the serum TSH level. In the presence of an intact hypothalamic/pituitary axis the serum TSH measurement is probably the most sensitive indicator of early primary hypothyroidism.

Under physiologic conditions synthesis and secretion of thyroid hormones are regulated extrathyroidally by TSH and intrathyroidally by intrinsic iodide metabolism. The autoregulation of thyroid hormone synthesis has recently been reviewed in some detail.[5] Of importance here are the following processes: First, serum iodide is concentrated in thyroid acinar cells by the so-called trapping mechanism. Through further synthetic pathways the inorganic iodide is rapidly organified to form monoiodotyrosine (MIT) and diiodotyrosine (DIT), precursors of thyroxine (T4) and triiodothyronine (T3). Iodide levels in the thyroid gland regulate the rate and extent of formation of precursor MIT and DIT as well as the products T4 and T3. By this means T4 and T3 synthesis is limited under physiologic conditions, and excessive secretion is prevented. These processes occur through what has been designated the Wolff-Chaikoff effect. This action of iodide is even more pronounced under pathologic conditions, and it may be responsible for the paradoxic ability of iodides to induce hypothyroidism or hyperthyroidism in certain goitrous conditions. Pharmacologic actions of iodides or thyroid hormone synthetic pathways are now well known, and it is important that they be appreciated in terms of thyroid hormone regulation, as well as in clinical therapy.

Several pathologic conditions can occur as a result of interference with the normal hypothalamic/pituitary/thyroid subsystem. The hyperthyroid syndromes related to thyrotropic excess may result from the extremely rare intrinsic excess of thyrotropic hormone or

Table 1-1
Etiologies of Different Thyrotoxic Syndromes

T4/T3 thyrotoxicosis

1. Graves' disease (diffuse toxic goiter with opthalmopathy)
2. Plummer's disease (toxic uninodular or multinodular goiter)
3. Thyrotoxicosis factitia (from desiccated thyroid, L-thyroxine, thyroglobulin, or liotrix)
4. Ectopic thyrotoxicosis (hydatidiform mole, choriocarcinoma, struma ovarii, metastatic thyroid cancer)
5. Thyrotropic thyrotoxicosis (TSH-secreting pituitary tumor)

T3 toxicosis

1. Nodular goiter with preferential T3 secretion
2. T3 toxicosis factitia (from liothyronine)
3. T3 toxicosis after radioactive iodine therapy for Graves' disease
4. Incipient thyrotoxicosis with T3 secretion

T4 toxicosis (?)

1. Syndromes of increased serum T4 with decreased serum T3 due to metabolic diversion to rT_3[12-16,20,21]

Table 1-2
Etiologies of Hypothyroid Syndromes

Primary hypothyroidism

    A. Nongoitrous hypothyroidism
      1. Idiopathic atrophy, congenital (cretinous) or adult
      2. Thyroiditis, subacute (rare) or chronic
      3. Postoperative
      4. Postradiation
    B. Goitrous hypothyroidism
      1. Hereditary (six types)
      2. Acquired
        a. Iodide myxedema
        b. Drug-induced hypothyroidism
        c. Chronic lymphoid (Hashimoto's) thyroiditis

Secondary hypothyroidism

    A. Anterior pituitary (Sheehan's, Simmonds') hypothyroidism
      1. Primary atrophy
      2. Tumors, granulomata, cysts, vascular events
      3. Pituitary ablation
    B. Hypothalamic hypothyroidism
      1. Granulomatous disorders
      2. TRH deficiencies
      3. Pituitary stalk section

Table 1–3
Some Differential Aspects of Hypothyroidism

Etiology	Serum TSH	Clinical Presentation
Primary hypothyroidism		
Thyroiditis, chronic	Elevated	Goiter with fibrous quality
Iatrogenic	Elevated	History of hyperthyroidism and treatment
Congenital errors of metabolism	Elevated	Family history of goiter; hypothyroidism at young age
Secondary hypothyroidism		
Idiopathic pituitary failure	Decreased	Loss of other pituitary hormones
Tumors	Decreased	Headaches, change in vision
Granulomas	Decreased	Signs and symptoms of sarcoid tuberculosis, etc.
Ischemic necrosis of pituitary (Sheehan's syndrome)	Decreased	Usually after parturition or severe hypertensive episode
Hypothalamic	Decreased (TRH stimulation test positive)	Rare causes other pituitary hormone deficiencies; occasionally associated with diabetes insipidus; may occur after parturition

more commonly from ectopic TSH syndromes (Graves' disease, molar thyrotoxicosis) or from autonomous thyroid gland secretion (Table 1–1). Hypothalamic, pituitary, and primary thyroid gland failures, from whatever etiologies (Table 1–2), result in hypothyroidism. If the cause of hypothyroidism is hypothalamic, TRH stimulation should reveal intact anterior pituitary function, as evidenced by an increase in serum TSH. On the other hand, anterior pituitary failure or inertia will be evidenced by low serum TSH levels as well as by the absence of, or a temporal delay in, the usual rise following TRH administration. Primary thyroid gland failure (by far the most common cause of hypothyroidism) is characterized generally by decreased serum FT4/FT3 concentrations and elevated serum TSH levels (> 10 μU/ml). By appropriate selection and interpretation of a few tests, most syndromes of primary, secondary (pituitary), or tertiary (hypothalamic) hypothyroidism can readily be identified (Tables 1–2 and 1–3).

Thyroid Hormone Transport in the Circulation

Thyroid gland secretion of T4 and T3 into the systemic circulation generally occurs as a steadily modulated process under TSH control, since only minute amounts of thyroid hormones are secreted in the absence of hypothalamic/pituitary stimulation. Once in the circulation, T4 and T3 are bound principally to serum thyroid binding globulin (TBG). Only T4 is weakly bound to a secondary carrier protein, designated thyroxine binding prealbumin (TBPA), and small quantities of both T4 and T3 are nonspecifically bound to serum albumin. The major portions of both T4 and T3 are thus bound in a dissociable complex with circulating proteins. Approximately 99.96 percent of T4 is bound, with 0.04 percent remaining free, whereas for T3, 99.6 percent is bound and about 0.4 percent

Table 1-4
Factors Altering Serum TBG Concentrations

Condition Increased serum TBG	T4D	TBG Binding Sites*	FT4
Pregnancy	▲	▼	N
Newborn infants	▲	▼	N
Estrogens (medication, tumors)	▲	▼	N
Congenital TBG excess	▲	▼	N
Decreased serum TBG			
Androgens	▼	▲	N
Nephrosis	▼	▲	N
Cirrhosis	▼	▲	N
Malnutrition, major illness	▼	▲	N
Salicylates	▼	▲	N
Hydantoins	▼	N/▲	N
Glucocorticoids	▼	▲	N
Congenital TBG deficiency		▲	N

*Dialyzable fraction (DF) or resin T3 uptake ratio (RT 3R) measurements.

▲ = increased; ▼ = decreased; N = normal; N/▲ = normal or increased; N/▼ = normal or decreased.

remains free. The larger portion of T3 remaining free, its greater intercellular binding, and its greater metabolic potency as compared to that of T4 appear to account for the observation that T3 produces roughly 50 percent of normal thyroid hormone thermogenic activity.

It is now generally appreciated that despite the larger quantities of T4 and T3 bound to serum proteins it is the minute quantities of free T4 (FT4) and free T3 (FT3) that best reflect the tissue metabolic activities of these hormones. The total serum concentrations of T4 and T3 are dependent on two major factors: the total amount of serum proteins available to bind T4 and T3 and the extent that these protein binding sites are saturated by T4 and T3. The amount of T4 or T3 bound to serum proteins affects only the total serum concentration of these hormones; it does not alter the concentration of FT4 or FT3. On the other hand, the extent of saturation of serum proteins by T4 or T3 directly alters the concentrations of FT4 and FT3 and consequently the tissue metabolic changes. An appreciation of these relationships is important; they are reviewed in detail in a number of currently available publications.[1-5,10,11] The major factors that alter the concentration of serum thyroid binding proteins are listed in Table 1-4. Increases in only serum TBG levels result in a new equilibrium state, which in euthyroid subjects causes an increase in the total serum T4 or T3 concentration and a decrease in the proportion (fraction) of total T4 or T3 that is free (free fraction) and thus a normal concentration of FT4 or FT3. In contrast, alterations in the saturation of available binding sites on TBG result in distinct changes in the concentration of FT4 or FT3. It is thus critical to the interpretation of serum thyroid hormone levels to appreciate these two important factors: the quantity of TBG in the serum and the degree of saturation of this TBG by T4 or T3. With this information the concentrations of FT4 and FT3 are derived by mathematical calculation:

$$FT4 = total\ T4 \times free\ fraction\ T4$$
$$FT3 = total\ T3 \times free\ fraction\ T3$$

The serum T4 is derived solely from thyroid gland secretions under physiologic conditions. This is not true for the serum T3, which is synthesized, in part, in the thyroid gland and is derived to a somewhat greater extent from tissue catabolic deiodination of T4. It is now appreciated that under a wide variety of conditions the catabolic deiodination of T4 to T3 is modified such that a disproportion in the serum ratio of T4 to T3 occurs. Such factors as age,[12] chronic illness[13,14] or surgery,[15] protein-caloric malnutrition,[16] drugs,[17] and the endogenous synthesis and secretion of T3 by the thyroid gland (T3 toxicosis) significantly alter both the total and free T3 levels in serum and their relationships to the total and free T4. It is thus prudent for diagnostic purposes to rely more critically on the total and free T4 levels, except in a few uncommon clinical conditions. Despite an active argument to the contrary,[18,19] it is prudent to continue to presume that both FT4 and FT3 are metabolically active thyroid hormones capable of the same qualitative calorigenic actions. When there is a disproportionate serum ratio of T4 to T3, it is the sum of the thermogenic potencies of the T4/T3 package that reflects tissue hormonal activity, rather than the concentration of either free hormone alone.

Recently a new metabolic pathway for T4 deiodination has been identified, in addition to the more active product 3,5,3'-triiodothyronine. This is 3,3',5'-triiodothyronine (reverse T3), a metabolically weak or inactive catabolite. In some clinical situations the T4-to-T3 pathway is diverted to excessive formation of reverse T3.[12,13,15,20,21] This will be discussed further in a later section.

Peripheral Tissue Actions of Thyroid Hormones

Despite the recent renewed interest in the manner by which thyroid hormones affect cellular and intracellular biochemical processes,[19,22] the exact mechanisms and pathways of thyroid hormones at the subcellular level remain enigmatic. Of the several concepts proposed, the most intriguing is the relationship of thyroid hormones (which are amino acids derived from iodotyrosines) to biogenic amine metabolism. The interaction of thyroid hormones in catecholamine regulation of neurohumoral functions is currently under investigation.[23] At present, the best laboratory measurement for evaluation of the effects of thyroid hormones on tissue metabolic processes is the serum FT4 and secondarily (in appropriate circumstances) the serum FT3.[24,25] However, clinical determination of the overall metabolic status of the patient is still the most reliable parameter on which to base clinical appraisals. The indirect tests of tissue thyroid hormone actions [basal metabolic rate (BMR), cholesterol, photomotography, enzymes, systolic time intervals,[26] etc.] may be useful in assisting in this appraisal, but they now play only a small role in the broad evaluation of thyroid functional status.

COMMONLY USED LABORATORY TESTS OF THYROID FUNCTION

In daily practice, identifying the site of a particular aberration in thyroid (metabolic) function is predicated primarily on sound clinical appraisal of the patient, which includes a thorough history and a careful physical examination. The vast majority of patients with overt forms of thyroidal dysfunction are identifiable on clinical grounds alone. Perhaps less than 10 percent require involved or uncommonly used tests for appropriate diagnosis. Fortunately, laboratory resources are now available to permit accurate and precise evaluation of the majority of patients with disorders of thyroid function; with appropriate in-

Table 1–5
Clinical Laboratory Tests for Appraisal of Thyroid Function

Hypothalamic/pituitary/thyroid relationships
1. Thyroidal radioiodine uptake and suppression tests
2. Thyrotropin (TSH) and thyrotropin releasing hormone (TRH) provocative tests
3. Serum immunoreactive TSH levels (IR-TSH)
4. Tests for intrathyroidal synthetic pathways

Circulating thyroid hormone levels
1. Serum total thyroxine (T4) concentration
   a. Chemical iodine methods: PBI, BEI, T4I; T4D (Murphy-Pattee); immunoreactive T4 (IR-T4)
2. Serum total triiodothyronine levels
   a. Immunoreactive T3 (IR-T3); immunoreactive reverse T3 (IR-rT3)
3. Serum TBG saturation
   a. Dialyzable fraction of T4 or T3 (DF); resin T3 uptake, resin T4 uptake, etc.
4. Free thyroxine concentration or index
   a. T4D $\times$ DF (T4) = (T4) = free T4 concentration (FT4); T4D $\times$ RT3 (ratio) = free T4 index (FTI-RT3)
5. Free triiodothyronine concentration
   a. IR-T3 $\times$ DF (T3) = free T3 concentration (FT3)

Tissue oxidative metabolism
1. Basal metabolic rate (BMR)
2. Serum cholesterol, enzymes creatine phosphokinase, lactic dehydrogenase
3. Electrocardiogram, Achilles tendon reflex
4. Clinical appraisal: skin, hair, pulse, etc.

terpretation these tests will provide the physician with excellent confirmatory measurements. The major disadvantages in regard to the numerous diagnostic tests in current use relate to excessive reliance on single determinations (technicians and applied technology are not infallible) and, more important, misinterpretation of accurate laboratory results. It is a good axiom to follow that when there is discordance between the laboratory results (or interpretation) and the clinical appraisal a further effort should be made to identify the reason for the incongruence, either by repeated tests or by use of other laboratory measurements for verification.

In actual practice, since thyroidal dysfunction generally follows common patterns, only a few well-selected tests are necessary to corroborate the clinical diagnosis in the majority of instances. These are listed in Table 1-5 and are discussed briefly in the following sections.

Tests of Hypothalamic/Pituitary/Thyroid Function

It is generally useful to apply the most specific tests available to derive the most useful information possible. Once the clinical impression is determined as to the most likely site of origin of hormonal dysfunction, the following tests are useful to confirm and delineate the biochemical pattern.

HYPOTHYROIDISM

The majority of patients with hypothyroidism exhibit the primary variety: that is, failure of the thyroid gland to secrete sufficient thyroid hormones to sustain tissue euthyroidism. The most common causes (Table 1–2) are chronic lymphoid thyroiditis (goitrous hypothyroidism) and ablative procedures (thyroidectomy, radioactive iodine). The characteristic pattern of serum thyroid hormones when the serum TBG levels are normal (Table 1–G) is a low T4 concentration (< 3.5 μg/dl), a low measure of serum free T4 fraction [resin T3 uptake ratio (RT3R) < 0.80] a low FT4 (calculated as T4 times RT3R), and, most important, a high serum TSH as measured by radioimmunoassay (TSH-RIA). The serum TSH-RIA is generally greater than 10 μU/ml by most assay methods. The serum T3 radioimmunoassay (T3-RIA) is also usually low, but not invariably so (the lower limit of normal is about 90 mg/dl). The serum T3-RIA in hypothyroidism can be within normal limits, with a low T4 and an increased TSH. The older nonspecific tests (BMR, cholesterol, enzymes, creatine tolerance, photomotography) can be supportive to the clinical appraisal, but they are not to be relied on for diagnostic discrimination (Table 1–5). The serum iodine determinations (PBI, BEI, T4I) have now been replaced by the more specific radioassays for T4 (T4D, thyroxine by displacement analysis, Murphy-Pattee; T4-RIA, radioimmunoassay for T4). These latter measurements are commonly available and are to be preferred for their specificity, precision, and reliability (Table 1–6).

Three clinical variants of the foregoing laboratory patterns in hypothyroidism are important. The first occurs with a low serum T4 concentration, a low free T4 fraction (RT3R), and a low FT4 calculation, but a low (rather than high) serum TSH level (usually < 1 μU/ml). This variant is a clue to the possibility of anterior pituitary insufficiency (pituitary hypothyroidism) or, on rare occasions, hypothalamic hypothyroidism.[27] Hypothalamic and pituitary hypothyroidism are critical diagnoses requiring confirmation, since initiation of thyroid hormone therapy prior to glucocorticoid replacement could precipitate adrenal (addisonian) crisis. In postmenopausal women a serum immunoreactive FSH determination can be useful in this differentiation.

The second variant is more commonly encountered in clinical practice, and on first observation it is quite confusing. This results from alterations in serum TBG levels (Table 1–4) along with associated hypothyroidism. The more commonly encountered syndrome is observed with increased serum TBG as a consequence of estrogen therapy (contraceptive pills). With primary hypothyroidism and increased serum TBG the serum T4 concentration is often in the low normal range (rather than distinctly low), and the free T4 fraction test (RT3R), which is low (as in hypothyroidism with normal TBG), does not correct fully the serum T4 value. Thus the calculated FT4 is frequently in the low normal range (rather than truly low). Similarly, the serum total T3 value, like the T4, might also be low normal (despite hypothyrodism) from the increased TBG. The major diagnostic determinant in this situation is the serum TSH level. This is high in primary hypothyroidism, since the true values for FT4 and FT3 are actually (but not by these tests) low. A careful history usually elicits use of an estrogen-containing medication. A comparable but somewhat different pattern is also noted occasionally with low serum TBG concentrations due to a variety of causes (Table 1–4). In this situation the patient is clinically euthyroid, but the serum T4 value is low as a result of low serum TBG levels or because of diversion of T3 to reverse T3.[21] In contrast to the situation where hypothyroidism is present, low TBG levels in euthyroid patients result in an increased free

Table 1-6
Representative Values for Some Useful Tests of Thyroid Function

Clinical Status	T4D (µg/dl)	DF (% ± SD)	FT4 (ng/dl)	RT3 (ratio)	FT4 Ix (RT3)	IR-T3 (ng/dl)	IR-TSH (µU/ml)
Euthyroidism	4–11.0	0.038 ± 0.004	1.5–3.3	0.95–1.15	4.5–10.5	80–190	< 8.0
Borderline low Hypothyroidism	3–4.0 < 3.0	0.030 ± 0.004	> 1.5	0.8–0.95 0.5–0.8	3.4–4.5 < 3.5	< 80	8–12.0 > 12.0
Borderline high Thyrotoxicosis	10–12.0 > 12.0	0.075 ± 0.031	3.3	1.15–1.26 > 1.26	10.5–12.5 > 12.5	> 190	< 2.0 < 1.0
Pregnancy	5–14.0	0.027 ± 0.006	1.5–3.3	0.5–0.95	2.6–11.3	100–250	< 8.0

Table 1-7
Some Clinical Conditions Resulting in Discordant Serum T4: T3 Ratios

	Serum T4*	Serum T3*
1. Synthetic thyroid hormone therapy		
a. levothyroxine	▲	N/▲
b. liothyronine	▼	▲
2. Iodide deficiency (severe)	▼	N
3. Post radioactive iodine therapy	▼	N/▲
4. Post antithyroid drug therapy	▼	N
5. Old age, chronic illness	N/▼	▼
6. Neonatal life (at birth)	▲	▼
7. After TSH stimulation	N	▲

*▲ = increased; ▼ = decreased; N = normal; N/▲ = normal or increased; N/▼ = normal or decreased.

T4 fraction (RT3R), but this frequently may be of insufficient magnitude to correct the serum T4 value into the normal FT4 range. A similar finding occurs in these circumstances with the serum T3 level.[14] As in the previous example, the factitiously low value for the FT4 or FT3 can be challenged by obtaining a serum TSH level; if it is increased, this would indicate primary hypothyroidism. If the serum TSH value is normal or low, this does not rule out pituitary or hypothalamic hypothyroidism. If this latter possibility exists, a TRH stimulation test will determine which of the two possible etiologies is responsible. If pituitary hypothyroidism is the cause, the serum TSH response to TRH will be absent. If hypothalamic hypothyroidism exists,[27] the serum TSH response to TRH will be significant. A serum immunoreactive FSH determination can also be useful in this differential diagnosis.

The third variant of the usual serum pattern in primary hypothyroidism occurs in the presence of physiologic doses of thyroid replacement therapy with synthetic thyroid hormones or in patients with divergent ratios of serum T4 to serum T3 (Table 1-7). In the former instance, patients or replacement dosages of L-thyroxine (250–350 mg/day) usually exhibit increased serum T4 concentrations, with elevated values of the free T4 fraction tests (RT3R, etc.) and increased FT4 values despite clinical euthyroidism. The exact reason for this is now unclear, in view of recent studies indicating that a large portion of serum T4 is deiodinated catabolically to serum T3.[28] The other etiology of this pharmacologic effect results from liothyronine replacement therapy (75–100 μg/day) in hypothyroid or euthyroid subjects. In this situation the pattern is a low value for serum T4 concentration (usually 1.0 μg/dl) but normal values for the free T4 fraction tests (RT3R, etc.). The calculated FT4 is thus still in the low range, despite full euthyroidism. The serum TSH levels would be low in both the above situations as a physiologic result of euthyroidism. The serum T3 levels are usually normal to high normal with levothyroxine therapy and quite high (especially during the first hour or so) after ingestion of liothyronine.

It is not generally appreciated that tests to measure the free T4 fraction (RT3R, etc) do not fully currect the serum T4 concentration when extremely high or low levels of serum TBG occur.[2,29] This is caused by finite upper and lower limits for these tests, which are valid only with moderate alterations in serum TBG levels. Similarly, with synthetic thyroid hormones used singly (levothyroxine or liothyronine), the FT4 value is also not valid. And lastly, for similar reasons, the FT4 calculation may not be accurate if the usual serum ratio of T4 to T3 is distorted. This occurs in T3 toxicosis, in iodide deficiency (chronic), following radioiodine therapy for thyrotoxicosis, and occasionally after abrupt cessation of antithyroid drugs in thyrotoxicosis or administration of TSH to normal or goitrous subjects (Table 1–7). For the above reasons it is important to appreciate that recently marketed testing kits that provide only values for measurements of FT4 without generating values for serum T4 and free T4 fraction (RT3R, etc.) will not give any indication of the reason for spuriously high or low results in the FT4 determination.

HYPERTHYROIDISM

The hypothalamic/pituitary solidus thyroid abnormality that is present in hyperthyroidism requires some clarification in light of recent developments. First, it is useful to differentiate the terms hyperthyroidism and thyrotoxicosis, despite the interchangeability of these terms in common usuage. *Hyperthyroidism* can be defined as that abnormality of thyroid gland function that results from ectopic or intrinsic (nonphysiologic) excess stimulation of secretion of thyroid hormones. This occurs as a result of ectopic thyrotropins (LATS, molar thyrotropin, or excess HCG) or from autonomous thyroid gland hypersecretions (''hot'' nodules, rare metastatic thyroid carcinomas). Under these circumstances the thyroid gland is no longer under physiologic regulation by the TRH/TSH mechanism, and the hypothalamic/pituitary centers are fully inhibited by the takeover of the ectopic mechanism. On the other hand, the term *thyrotoxicosis* implies excessive stimulation of tissue oxidative (thyrothermogenic) processes by increased tissue availability of thyroid hormones. This may occur from either endogenous or exogenous sources or from either or both thyroid hormones in varying ratios (Table 1–1). In hyperthyroidism the thyroid gland synthetic pathways are operating at supranormal rates, usually but not always accompanied by excessive secretions of thyroid hormones (thyrotoxicosis). Less commonly, hyperthyroidism can be associated with normal thyroid secretions and euthyroidism (ophthalmic Graves' disease and nonsuppressible ''hot'' nodules) and on rare occasions even with hypothyroidism (Table 1–8). The laboratory assessment for determining hyperthyroidism, for the most part, has been the so-called suppression test. By administering exogenous thyroid hormones for 5–10 days and using the radioiodine uptake test[30] or serum T4 changes[11,31] as objective determinants, the integrity of the hypothalamic/pituitary/thyroid axis is definable. Generally, radioiodine uptake values above 20 percent in 24 hr after a week or more of full replacement doses of thyroid hormones indicate hyperthyroidism. A more recent approach to this diagnosis involves the serum TSH response to exogenous TRH stimulation. Failure of the serum TSH to rise indicates refractoriness or inertia of the pituitary gland because of prior ''priming'' by a hyperfunctioning thyroid gland or because of exogenous thyroid hormones in both physiologic and pharmacoloogic dosages[11,31]

It is now possible to localize the intrathyroidal sites where abnormalities of synthesis have occurred. The iodide-perchlorate test is useful in determining the most common locus, which occurs at the step in iodide organification to form iodotyrosines.[33] The interested reader is referred to more detailed reviews.[9,34,35]

Table 1–8
"Hashitoxicosis" with Hypothyroidism*

Test	2-19-73	2-27-73	Normal Range
Radioiodine uptake	46%		15%–40%
T3 suppression test (100 μg/day liothyronine)		27%	<20%
Serum values			
T4	2.6 μg/dl	2.2 μg/dl	4–11
RT4 ratio	0.86 μg/dl	0.95 μgdl	0.80–1.25
Total IR-T3	139 ng/dl	543 ng/dl	90–180
IR-TSH	>80 μU/ml	<10 μU/ml	0–8
Thyroglobulin antibodies	1:2,560	1:2,560	<1:80

*56-year-old female patient presenting with unilateral exophthalmos.

Tests of Thyroid Hormone Transport in the Circulation

The most commonly used tests of thyroid metabolic function are those that measure the concentrations of total serum TBG-bound T4 and T3, along with some relative measure of the quantities of the free moieties FT4 and FT3. It is now well appreciated that the major portion of the serum total T4 circulates as a dissociable complex with TBG but that only FT4 and FT3 correlate with the tissue activity of these hormones. Thus, when the combined metabolic potential of serum FT4 and FT3 is consistent with euthyroidism (regardless of the relationship of FT4 to FT3), the patient is considered euthyroid. Recent information indicates that the usual serum ratio of FT4 to FT3 of approximately 5:1 varies considerably, depending on a number of factors (Table 1–7). T3 toxicosis is an example of discordant FT4:FT3 ratios in thyrotoxicosis, and examples of T3 euthyroidism (where FT4 is normal but FT3 is very low) have been described. The use of total and free T3 alone as diagnostic discriminators is considered inaccurate generally, except for the diagnosis of thyrotoxicosis.

SERUM TOTAL T4 AND FREE T4

The classic use of serum iodine measurement as an indicator of total serum T4 concentration (PBI, BEI, T4I, etc.) has recently been replaced by radioassay procedures. More commonly, the serum T4 by displacement radioassay (T4D) is generally used, with the usual normal range of 4.0 – 11.0 μg/dl. The serum T4 by radioimmunoassay (T4-RIA) is based on a comparable technique and gives roughly the same normal range. It is important to appreciate that these assays are not totally specific for L-thyroxine, since they will also measure serum D-thyroxine (Choloxin). The designation T4I was applied originally to a process to alter the T4D result to a value comparable to the PBI result by taking 65% of the T4D (the molecular content of iodine). This value no longer has any clinical utility, and it should be discarded.

To most physicians the method of calculating FT4 is confusing. In simple terms, serum total T4 is a true indicator of FT4 only when the serum TBG concentration is normal. Thus when serum TBG is high or low, the serum T4 value does not correspond to the FT4. By multiplying the serum T4 by a factor that accounts for the change in serum TGB quantitatively, a new value for serum T4 is obtained that is proportionate to FT4. This has been termed the FT4 index or FT4 Ix. The more technically complex method of applying this correction factor is to obtain a dialyzable fraction for free T4 and then multiply it by the total serum T4 concentration to obtain FT4. In clinical practice comparable but less precise and less inclusive methods are used. These are generally termed particulate binding tests, with the resin T3 uptake test (RT3) being the most commonly used. These are discussed in detail elsewhere.[2,5,11] It should be reemphasized here that the resin T3 and resin T4 uptake tests use T3 and T4 only as binding reagents and that they measure only the available binding sites on serum TBG, not serum T3 and T4! Second, their ability to correct serum total T4 for alterations in TBG is limited, since these tests have finite upper and lower limits and thus are not accurate when extreme changes in serum TBG are encountered. Lastly, since they measure available binding sites on TBG, other substances that are bound to TBG give spurious results (dextrothyroxine, levothyroxine, salicylates, hydantoins, etc.). Use of these tests alone for thyroid diagnosis is not justified in view of their many limitations. They serve best as measurements with which to derive the FT4 index from the serum total T4. The resin T3 uptake should be expressed as a ratio of a standard reference serum in order to compensate for interassay variations and for simplicity of calculating FT4.[36]

SERUM TOTAL T3 AND FT3 CONCENTRATIONS

The development of a sensitive and precise radioimmunoassay for serum T3 measurements has been of great value in clarifying our understanding of this potent thyroid hormone. However, its impact on clinical diagnosis is still limited by its metabolic uniqueness: the rapid entrance and egress of T3 from the circulation and its rapid dissociation from binding to TBG. The usual range for serum total T3 concentration is 80–190 ng/dl (Table 1–6), but this varies in different laboratories because of differing techniques. The more useful, but as yet unstandardized, method for obtaining FT3 concentration is by use of dialysis techniques for T3 similar to but more difficult than that for T4. The use of the resin T3 uptake ratio to correct the total T3 for TBG alterations appears to provide an approximate correlation with the FT3 obtained by dialysis. At the present time the T3-RIA is employed clinically to diagnose T3 thyrotoxicosis and to identify other varieties of clinical syndromes where the ratio of FT4 to FT3 differs from the normal range. The previously identified problems in interpreting the serum T3 concentrations in clinical diagnosis should be appreciated. In addition, the serum T3 determination should be drawn at least 12–24 hr after ingestion of liothyronine or liotrix to permit time for systemic equilibration. Otherwise, factitiously high levels will be reported because of rapid absorption of T3; these levels are not reflective of the tissue metabolic status of the patient. Despite the rapid rise and fall of serum total T3 concentrations after ingestion of T3-containing preparations, the metabolic effects of this rise are not reflected metabolically or in rapid TSH fluctuations,[37] probably because the major portion of the recently absorbed T3 is bound to TBG.

THYROID HORMONE METABOLITES, CONGENERS, AND ISOMERS

It was previously noted that interpretation of serum levels of total T4 and T3 must be regarded carefully in the context of existing serum ratios of T4 to T3 and of serum TBG concentrations. In addition, careful attention to other substances that bind to serum TBG is necessary to avoid misinterpretation of these tests. These include drugs (salicylates, hydantoins, etc.), thyroid hormone isomers (dextrothyroxine), and congeners (which are not available for clinical use such as alkyl, halogen, or side-chain congeners, as well as derivatives). A recent and exciting discovery is the metabolite of T3 known as reverse T3 (rT3). This reverse triiodothyronine (3,3',5'-L-triiodothyronine) is one of the two catabolic metabolites of 3,5,3',5'-L-thyroxine. Under some conditions, as previously discussed, T4 is apparently preferentially deiodinated to reverse T3, which is calorigenically inert.[38] At the present time, awareness of this metabolite is important in the evaluation of the neonate[20] and in certain clinical states.[12,13,15,21]

Tests of Peripheral Actions of Thyroid Hormones

Since the application of oxygen spirometry to the diagnosis of thyrotoxicosis by Magnus-Levy in 1895, several tests have been devised that utilize some action of thyroid hormones on tissue oxidative processes. These include the BMR, serum cholesterol, enzymes, creatine tolerance, sleeping pulse rate, ECG changes, Achilles tendon reflex, etc. All are nonspecific and are modified by nonthyroidal conditions and diseases. Of particular interest has been the role of catecholamine metabolism in thyroid hormone action, and some recent information bears critically on this fascinating relationship.[39] It is not generally appreciated that one of the earliest tests of thyroid function employed the response to epinephrine administration (Goetsch test). The recent introduction into clinical practice of β-adrenergic blocking agents, particularly propranolol, has provided a group of potent antagonists to the peripheral actions of excessive thyroid hormones. These agents interfere with the catecholamine actions of thyroid hormones without altering the oxidative metabolism of serum thyroid hormone concentrations.

With the current widespread availability of precise and accurate measurements of thyroid function, the nonspecific tests such as the BMR no longer have a useful place in the physician's diagnostic armamentarium. However, this does not negate evaluation of the tissue effects of thyroid hormones under a wide variety of clinical circumstances. This can best be evaluated by a careful clinical examination, with particular emphasis on tissue alterations, which are well described in general textbooks. There is no substitute for a clinical evaluation and the carefully evolved judgments that are derived therefrom. These are the cornerstones of sound medical practice. Laboratory tests, no matter how carefully obtained and determined, are only adjuncts to the physician's careful and objective evaluation of the patient's status. More errors will be made by unquestioned reliance on the results of laboratory tests than by reliance on sound clinical judgment.

REFERENCES

1. Werner SC, Ingbar SH (eds): The Thyroid. A Fundamental and Clinical Text (ed 3). New York, Harper & Row, 1971
2. Selenkow HA: The Normal and Abnormal Thyroid. An Approach to Diagnosis and Therapy. New York, Medcom Press, 1973
3. Brown J (moderator): Thyroid physiology in health and disease (UCLA conference). Ann Intern Med 81:68–81, 1974
4. Burrow GN (ed): Current concepts of thyroid disease (symposium). Med Clin North Am 59:1043–1275, 1975
5. Selenkow HA, Himathongkam T: Thyroid disease in adolescence: Diagnosis and therapy, in Gallagher JR, Heald FP, Garell DC (eds): Medical Care of the Adolescent (ed 3). New York, Appleton-Century-Crofts, 1975
6. Carlson HE, Hershman JM: The hypothalamic-

pituitary-thyroid axis. Med Clin North Am 59:1045–1053, 1975
7. Chopra IJ, Chopra U, Orgiazzi J: Abnormalities of hypothalamic-hypophyseal-thyroid axis in patients with Graves' opthalmopathy. J Clin Endocrinal Metab 37:955–967, 1973
8. Stahl TJ: Radioimmunoassay and the hormones of thyroid function. Semin Nucl Med 5:221–246, 1975
9. Vagenakis AG, Braverman LE: Adverse effects of iodides on thyroid function. Med Clin North Am 59:1075–1088, 1975
10. Selenkow HA, Newmark SR: Thyroidal dysfunction: Diagnosis and therapy. Primary Care 1:23–44, 1974
11. Selenkow HA: Clinical laboratory appraisal of thyroid function, in Behrman SJ, Kistner RW (eds): Progress in Infertility. Boston, Little, Brown, 1975
12. Britton KE, Ellis SM, Miralles JM, et al: Is "T4 toxicosis" a normal biochemical finding in elderly? Lancet 2:141–142, 1975
13. Carter JN, Corcoran JM, Eastman CJ, et al: Effect of severe, chronic illness on thyroid dysfunction. Lancet 2:971–974, 1974
14. Bernudez F, Surks MI, Oppenheimer JH: High incidence of decreased serum triiodothyronine concentrations in patients with nonthyroidal disease. J Clin Endocrinol Metab 41:27–40, 1975
15. Burr WA, Black EG, Griffiths RS, et al: Serum triiodothyronine and reverse triiodothyronine concentrations after surgical operations. Lancet 2:1277–1279, 1975
16. Vagenakis AG, Burger A, Portnay GI, et al: Diversion of peripheral thyroxine metabolism from activating to inactivating pathways during complete fasting. J Clin Endocrinol Metab 41:191–194, 1975
17. Oppenheimer JH, Schwartz HL, Surks MI: Propylthiouracil (PTU) inhibits the conversion of L-thyroxine (T4) to L-triiodothyronine (T3): A possible explanation of the anti-T4 effect of PTU and further support of the concept that T3 is the primary thyroid hormone. J Clin Invest 51:2493-F, 1972
18. Chopra IJ, Solomon DH, Chua Teco GN: Thyroxine: Just a prohormone or a hormone too? J Clin Endocrinol Metab 36:1050–1057, 1973
19. Oppenheimer JH, Surks MI: The peripheral action of the thyroid hormones. Med Clin North Am 59:1055–1061, 1975
20. Chopra IJ, Sack J, Fisher DA: Reverse T3 in the fetus and newborn, in Fisher DA, Burrow GN (eds): Perinatal Thyroid Physiology and Disease. New York, Raven Press, 1975
21. Chopra IJ, Chopra U, Smith SR, et al: Reciprocal changes in serum concentrations of 3,3',5'-triiodothyronine (reverse T3), 3,5,3'-triiodothyronine (T3) in systemic illness. J Clin Endocrinol Metab 41:1043–1049, 1975
22. Sterling FH: Thyroxine pathways—hypothesis (letter to the editor). N Engl J Med 293:309, 1975
23. Dratman MB: On the mechanism of action of thyroxine, an amino acid analogue of tyrosine. J Theor Biol 46:255–270,1974
24. Larsen PR: Tests of thyroid function. Med Clin North Am 59:1063–1074, 1975
25. Shalet SM, Beardwell CG, Lamb SM et al: Value of routine serum-triiodothyronine estimation in diagnosis of thyrotoxicosis. Lancet 2:1008–1018, 1975
26. Parisi AF, Hamilton BP, Thomas CN, et al: Systolic time intervals in thyrotoxicosis. Circulation 49:900–904, 1974
27. Pittman JA, Haigler ED, Hershman JM, et al: Hypothalamic hypothyroidism. N Engl J Med 285:844–845, 1971
28. Utiger RD: Serum triiodothyronine in man. Ann Rev Med 25:289–302, 1974
29. Selenkow HA: Tests for circulating thyroid hormones, in Selenkow HA, Hoffman F (eds): Diagnosis and Treatment of Common Thyroid Diseases. Excepta Medica International Congress Series No 227, Amsterdam, Excerpta Medica, 1971
30. Burke G: The triiodothyroxine suppression test. Am J Med 42:600–609, 1967
31. Duick DA, Stein RB, Warren DW, et al: The significance of partial suppressibility of serum thyroxine by triiodothyronine administration in euthyroid man. J Clin Endocrinol Metab 41:229–234, 1975
32. Krugman LG, Hershman JM, Chopra IJ, et al: Patterns of recovery of the hypothalamic-pituitary-thyroid axis in patients taken off chronic thyroid therapy. J Clin Endocrinol Metab 41:70–80, 1975
33. Selenkow HA, Garcia AM, Bradley EB: An autoregulatory effect of iodide in diverse thyroid disorders. Ann Intern Med 62:714–726, 1965
34. Ingbar SH: Autoregulation of the thyroid response to iodide excess and depletion. Mayo Clin Proc 47:814–823, 1972
35. Stanbury JB, Wyngaarden JB, Fredrickson DS (eds): The Metabolic Basis of Inherited Disease (ed 3). New York, McGraw-Hill, 1972
36. Solomon DH, Benotti J, de Groot LJ, et al: Nomenclature for tests of thyroid hormones in serum: Report of a committee of the American Thyroid Association. J Clin Endocrinol Metab 34:884–890, 1972
37. Saberi M, Utiger RD: Serum thyroid hormone

and thyrotropin concentrations during thyroxine and triiodothyronine therapy. J Clin Endocrinol Metab 39:923–927, 1974
38. Pittman JA, Brown RW, Register HB Jr: Biological activity of 3,3',5'-triiodo-DL-thyronine. Endocrinology 70:79–83, 1962
39. Spaulding SW, Noth RH: Thyroid-catechol interactions. Med Clin North Am 59:1123–1131, 1975

Robert D. Utiger

2
Diagnosis and Treatment of Hypothyroidism

Hypothyroidism is the clinical expression of reduced thyroid hormone secretion; it responds to treatment with thyroid hormone. Its classic form, known as myxedema because of the clinical appearance and demeanor of the patient, is not difficult to recognize. However, its clinical manifestations are often more subtle, involving perhaps only one organ system or a few organ systems, so that recognition may be difficult. Hypothyroidism also may be defined in physiologic terms as reduced thyroid secretion that, when due to thyroid disease itself, is sufficient to activate the normal defense against thyroid deficiency, i.e., increased secretion of pituitary thyrotropin (TSH). Increased TSH secretion may correct the deficiency in thyroid hormone secretion to such an extent that few clinical manifestations of hypothyroidism are present. Hypothyroidism as defined in these terms is more frequent than the clinical form resulting from tissue thyroid hormone deficiency. From the practical point of view, hypothyroidism should be suspected when there are suggestive clinical manifestations (however mild or vague) or when goiter is present. Its diagnosis depends on recognition of its clinical manifestations, on awareness of its causes, and on use of confirmatory diagnostic tests. Because of the recent availability of more reliable diagnostic tests, the diagnosis of hypothyroidism can now be established in patients with mild or vague symptomatology with greater ease and certainty than was heretofore possible.

MANIFESTATIONS OF HYPOTHYROIDISM

Hypothyroidism results in the accumulation of glycosaminoglycans, primarily hyaluronic acid, in interstitial tissue. These substances are normal constituents of intercellular ground substance, and their accumulation in interstitial tissue in patients with hypothyroidism leads to the mucinous edema characteristic of this disorder. These changes are most clearly recognized in subcutaneous tissue, and mucinous edema there produces some of the most obvious clinical manifestations of hypothyroidism. In fatal cases mucinous edema is found in the interstitial tissue of many other organ systems, and it probably plays an important role in many of the functional abnormalities that accompany hypothyroidism.

Table 2-1
Major Causes of Hypothyroidism

Loss of functional thyroid tissue
    Idiopathic hypothyroidism
    Chronic autoimmune thyroiditis (Hashimoto's disease)
    Post ^{131}I therapy
    Thyroidectomy
    Thyroid dysgenesis

Thyroid biosynthetic defects
    Inherited defects
    Iodine deficiency
    Antithyroid agents

Hypothyrotropic Hypothyroidism
    TSH deficiency
    TRH deficiency

Peripheral Resistance to Thyroid Hormones

Thyroid hormone is required for normal functioning of virtually every organ system. If one term had to be chosen to apply to the functioning of most tissues in the presence of thyroid deficiency, it would be the term slowing. There is slowing of physical and mental activity and slowing of cardiovascular, gastrointestinal, and neuromuscular function. Common symptoms and signs are listed in Table 2–1.[1-4] Many of these also frequently occur in euthyroid patients. Certain symptoms, such as fatigue, lethargy, constipation, and dry skin or hair, are so common in other patients that their diagnostic value is limited. It has been found that the most discriminating symptoms and signs are delayed relaxation of ankle reflexes, slow movements, coarse skin, decreased sweating, hoarseness, paresthesias, cold intolerance, and periorbital edema.[5] Similar findings are seen in children with hypothyroidism, but in addition there is retardation of physical and mental development in infants less than 2 years of age. Since these effects may be permanent if hypothyroidism is not recognized and treated in the first months of life, this diagnosis must be considered in any infant with any of the signs of hypothyroidism and any degree of retardation.

Another factor that makes recognition of hypothyroidism difficult is the insidious onset and progression of the disease. Following thyroidectomy or abrupt withdrawal of thyroid hormone therapy in a hypothyroid patient, 3–4 weeks are required for the development of any symptoms, and overt hypothyroidism may not appear for many months.[6] This delay reflects the presence of substantial stores of thyroxine in extracellular fluid and certain tissues. Also, in most patients the onset of thyroid failure is not abrupt but develops over many months or years. As it progresses, each decline in thyroid secretion results in a further increase in TSH secretion, which may limit the decline in thyroid secretion and may even stabilize it if further thyroid damage does not occur.

The appearance of the patient with hypothyroidism may range from normal to overt myxedema. Often the major presenting manifestations are subjective. The patient complains of tiredness and weakness and cannot maintain normal activity. Attempts to elicit more specific symptoms or signs of hypothyroidism may fail; the patient either has not noted them or cannot remember. This behavior may be attributed to aging, either by the patient or by relatives. Cold intolerance may be marked, with the patient using extra clothing even in summer. As is often the case in endocrine disorders, however, compari-

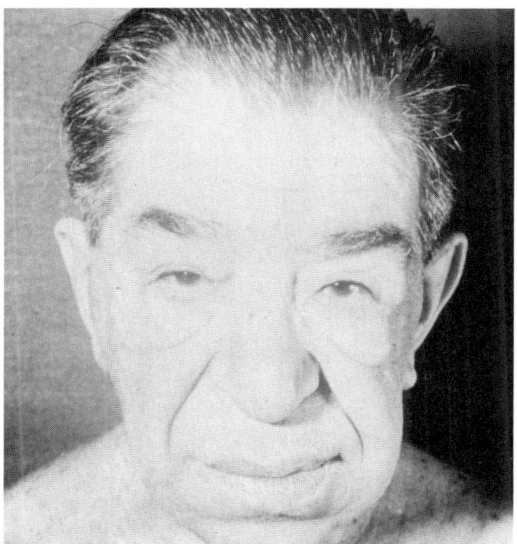

Fig. 2–1. Facial appearance of a patient with severe hypothyroidism. Note the marked periorbital edema.

son of pictures of the patient taken over a period of several years or questioning of relatives may provide clues to the diagnosis.

Skin and Appendages

The characteristic appearance of the patient with hypothyroidism reflects the effect of thyroid deficiency on the skin. The accumulation of mucinous edema results in nonpitting facial, periorbital, and peripheral edema involving both hands and feet. The facial features appear coarsened. Figure 2–1 shows a patient with marked facial features of hypothyroidism. Periorbital edema, an early finding, causes the edematous upper eyelid to droop and encroach on the pupil. There is hyperkeratosis of the epidermis, and the skin becomes rough, scaly, and thickened. More often the patient's appearance is less dramatically altered. The patient may complain of dry and scaly skin, but it is not thickened or particularly rough, and only mild periorbital and peripheral edema is present. At times the edema is pitting, particularly in the lower extremities, and such a finding does not indicate cardiac or other disease. There is often pallor, caused largely by thickening of the dermis and epidermis, by decreased cutaneous blood flow, and at times by anemia. Skin thickening and decreased blood flow also result in coldness of the skin. Decreased sebaceous and sweat gland secretions add to the dryness of the skin. The hair may become coarse, dry, and brittle with slowing or even cessation of hair growth.

Nervous System

Several manifestations of hypothyroidism relate to central nervous system dysfunction. These probably result from some degree of hypoxia, since brain glucose and oxygen consumption are not reduced, whereas cerebral vascular resistance is increased and cerebral blood flow is reduced by hypothyroidism.[7] Clinical features reflect slowing of many cerebral functions. These may be manifested only by complaints of tiredness, lethargy, and fatigue and by loss of ambition and energy. The patient becomes complacent and less aware of his surroundings. There is mental slowness and physical clumsiness. Speech is slow, hesitant, and hoarse. With the exception of memory loss, intellectual capacity is usually well preserved. The patient may describe significant limitation of activity with a trace of amusement, and such limitation may be accepted with equanimity. Hearing loss may be experienced. The patient may sleep longer at night or fall asleep frequently during the day. This may progress to almost constant somnolence and ultimately to coma, with hypothermia, respiratory depression, hypoglycemia, and/or water intoxication. Coma may occur spontaneously, or it may be coincident with the development of another illness or the result of inadvertent use of narcotics or analgesics.[8] Psychiatric manifestations of several types occur. Most often there is depression. Occasionally, dementia is marked, and rarely there is severe anxiety and agitation ("myxedema madness").

Hypothyroid patients often complain of paresthesias, but there are usually no objective neurologic findings. Several neurologic syndromes may occur. Perhaps the most frequent is the carpal tunnel syndrome: mucinous edema of the flexor retinaculum of the wrist resulting in median nerve compression. Other neurologic manifestations that may be present occasionally are polyneuropathy and cerebellar dysfunction, with signs such as ataxia, intention tremor, and nystagmus.[9]

Musculoskeletal System

The most characteristic abnormality in muscle function is the delay in relaxation time of the Achilles reflex (pseudomyotonia).[10] Muscle cramps and myalgias are frequent symptoms, and movements may be slow and clumsy. Subjective weakness and fatigability are common, but these and the slowness of movement are probably primarily manifestations of central nervous system dysfunction. Objective proximal muscle weakness does occur, however.[11] Hypothyroid patients may complain of vague articular pains and stiffness. There may be synovial and capsular thickening, with joint swelling and effusion, usually of the knees and small joints of the hands and feet.[12]

Cardiovascular-Pulmonary System

Thyroid hormones have direct effects on cardiac function; in their absence there is decreased rate and force of cardiac muscle contractibility.[13] Hypothyroidism also reduces oxygen requirements, and thus cardiac work is decreased. Peripheral resistance is increased, and cerebral, cutaneous, and renal blood flow and blood volume are reduced.[14] The physiologic consequence of these changes is decreased cardiac output due to decreases in heart rate and stroke volume. Clinical cardiovascular abnormalities in hypothyroid patients include bradycardia, signs of poor peripheral circulation (such as pallor and cold skin), sensitivity to cold, and hypertension. The heart sounds may be distant. Because of the lethargy, puffiness, edema, and diminished cardiac activity, these patients are often thought to have congestive heart failure. This is in fact rare, and digitalis therapy is of little benefit. Clinical and/or radiographic evidence of cardiac enlargement due to pericardial effusion and/or cardiac dilatation may be present. Pericardial effusion must occur slowly, since it is well tolerated and has little effect on cardiac dynamics. The electrocardiogram is often abnormal, most often showing bradycardia and low-amplitude P waves and QRS complexes. Serum creatine phosphokinase, glutamic oxaloacetic transaminase, and lactic dehydrogenase may be elevated.[15]

Hypercholesterolemia and hypertriglyceridemia occur in hypothyroidism frequently. Whether hypothyroidism results in accelerated atherogenesis is controversial, and data on this question are conflicting.[16,17] The development of hypothyroidism may ameliorate angina pectoris, possibly directly because cardiac work and myocardial oxygen requirements are reduced or possibly simply because the patient becomes less active.

There may be abnormalities in both the upper and the lower respiratory systems in hypothyroidism. Chronic nasal congestion due to mucinous edema of the nasal mucosa may be present. Hoarseness due to thickening of the vocal cords is common. Studies of pulmonary function have generally yielded fairly normal results. Lung volumes are normal. Vital capacity is normal, and arterial PO_2, PCO_2, and pH are maintained normally.[18] Maximum breathing capacity and compliance may be reduced. These changes reflect respiratory muscle weakness and/or respiratory center depression.

Renal Function

Serum concentrations of urea, creatinine, and electrolytes are normal, although there may be hyperuricemia due to decreased urate excretion. Plasma renin activity is decreased. Modest proteinuria and a modest defect in urine concentrating ability may be present. Hypothyroid patients may appear puffy, even edematous, and total body water and sodium are often increased. This results largely from sodium and water retention consequent to the extracellular glycosaminoglycan accumulation and is not consequent to impaired renal function. Occasionally hyponatremia with findings compatible with inappropriate vasopressin secretion are present, i.e., natriuresis and an increased urine/plasma osmolality ratio. It is not clear whether this is due to excess vasopressin production or to an intrinsic renal abnormality in water excretion.

Gastrointestinal System

Abnormalities in gastrointestinal function are common in hypothyroidism. The tongue is enlarged. Decreased gastric emptying and intestinal motility result in nausea, vomiting, abdominal distension, and constipation, particularly the latter. In some patients hypomotility may be so marked as to produce paralytic ileus or megacolon with the clinical picture of intestinal obstruction. A number of types of malabsorption are recognized. Gastric atrophy and achlorhydria are frequently present. In about 25 percent of patients with idiopathic hypothyroidism or chronic autoimmune thyroiditis, anti-parietal-cell antibodies are found. Defects in acid secretion and vitamin B_{12} malabsorption are frequent in patients with these types of hypothyroidism, and some either have or develop pernicious anemia.[19] Intestinal absorption of glucose and other sugars may be delayed or reduced, and rarely steatorrhea occurs.

Energy Metabolism

The major reduction in energy expenditure and oxygen consumption in hypothyroidism is accompanied by reduced utilization of a variety of substrates. These changes result in lessened heat production. Decreased metabolic activity and substrate utilization result in decreases in appetite and food intake. Body weight gain does occur; much of it is due to retention of salt and water rather than to tissue accumulation.

In general, patients with hypothyroidism maintain relatively normal carbohydrate metabolism, although glucose utilization is reduced. The glucose tolerance test curve is often flat because of delayed gastric emptying. Insulin responses to oral glucose are appropriate for the rise in glucose that occurs. In insulin-dependent diabetic patients exogenous insulin degradation is slowed, and thus insulin sensitivity may develop. Hypothyroid adults maintain positive nitrogen balance. There appears to be no abnormality in protein digestion or amino acid absorption or production.

Elevated plasma cholesterol concentrations are a common finding in thyroidal hypothyroidism, but not hypothyrotropic hypothyroidism. The major cause is decreased cholesterol metabolism and biliary excretion. Plasma triglyceride elevations also occur, but they are less frequent; rarely there is gross lipemia.[20]

Hematopoietic System

A common finding is a mild normocytic normochromic anemia, and reduction in red cell mass is even more frequent. The hemoglobin is rarely less than 10 g/dl. Erythropoietin levels are normal or low. The bone marrow is usually hypocellular, and kinetic studies indicate slowed iron clearance and incorporation. Serum iron, iron binding capacity, and vitamin B_{12} and folate concentrations are usually normal. These findings reflect adaptation to reduced peripheral oxygen consumption, and the reduced red cell mass does not reflect the presence of anemia.[21] Occasionally one of several types of deficiency anemia, with the appropriate peripheral blood and marrow findings, may be present. Thus iron deficiency may result from excessive menstrual bleeding and/or poor iron absorption secondary to decreased gastric acid production. Megaloblastic anemia may occur, caused either directly by thyroid hormone deficiency producing vitamin B_{12} malabsorption or by the presence of true pernicious anemia in patients with idiopathic hypothyroidism or chronic autoimmune thyroiditis.[19]

Endocrine System

Hypothyroidism may result in changes in pituitary and other endocrine gland functions. In some instances these changes reflect tropic hormone deficiencies occurring as a result of the hypothalamic or pituitary disease that causes the hypothyroidism. Other changes are the direct result of hypothyroidism. There is decreased turnover of cortisol, primarily a result of decreased hepatic steroid catabolism, and therefore excretion of urinary steroid metabolites is reduced.[22] Cortisol production is reduced. Plasma cortisol concentrations and urinary cortisol excretion remain normal. Pituitary-adrenal responses to metyrapone, hypoglycemia, and ACTH are normal in most patients.[23,24]

Gonadal steroid metabolism is similarly affected, there being a reduction in the overall rate of estradiol catabolism. Production of sex-hormone-binding globulin may be decreased. The consequences are reduced total estradiol concentrations, but free estradiol concentrations are normal or elevated. Serum follicle-stimulating hormone (FSH) and luteinizing hormone (LH) concentrations are usually in the normal nonovulatory range, although cyclic FSH and LH secretion may be interrupted.[25] The characteristic resultant abnormalities are anovulatory cycles and infertility. Menstrual bleeding may therefore become irregular and excessive, but occasionally amenorrhea results. In the male, plasma testosterone concentrations may be decreased due to reduced sex-hormone-binding globulin production, but serum free testosterone and gonadotropin concentrations are usually normal. There is little available information about reproductive capacity.

Growth hormone secretion in response to a variety of provocative stimuli such as hypoglycemia and arginine infusion is often reduced.[26] Basal serum prolactin concentra-

Table 2-2

Symptoms and Signs of Hypothyroidism*

Symptoms	Percentage of Patients
Dry Skin	62–97
Puffiness of hands, feet, face	40–90
Pallor	58–67
Thinning, dryness, or loss of hair	32–57
Sleepiness, tiredness	25–98
Lethargy, fatigue	25–95
Nervousness, anxiety	13–58
Slow speech	48–91
Impaired memory	48–66
Decreased reflexes	46
Hypertension	18
Bradycardia	8–14
Hoarseness	48–74
Weight gain	48–76
Constipation	38–61
Menstrual abnormalities	16–58

*Adapted from several large series.[1-4]

tions in most hypothyroid patients are in the normal range, but responses to stimuli such as thyrotropin releasing hormone are increased.[27] Rarely, prolactin secretion is increased and lactation occurs.[28]

CAUSES OF HYPOTHYROIDISM

Thyroid hormone synthesis and secretion involve a number of steps, and there are several extrathyroidal regulatory factors and an absolute requirement for iodine, which can be obtained only from the diet. Thus hypothyroidism may result from many different causes. A classification of causes is shown in Table 2-2.

The relative frequencies of the different forms of hypothyroidism are uncertain. In many areas iodine deficiency is still its most common cause. In the United States no recent figures are available, but in a study that was made a decade ago hypothyroidism was idiopathic in 40 percent of cases, and it followed ^{131}I therapy for hyperthyroidism in 20 percent of cases.[1] Today the proportion of patients with ^{131}I-induced hypothyroidism would probably be greater. While hypothyroidism occurs at all ages, it is most frequent after the fourth or fifth decade, and, as is true for most thyroid disorders, it is considerably more common in women.

Hypothyroidism Caused by Loss of Functional Thyroid Tissue

IDIOPATHIC HYPOTHYROIDISM (ATROPHIC THYROIDITIS)

Atrophy is one of the most frequent causes of hypothyroidism. It is most common in women after the fourth decade. The thyroid gland is recognizable only as a small remnant consisting of fibrous tissue and a few follicles, with varying degrees of lymphocytic infiltration.[29] These findings suggest prior thyroid destruction by an inflammatory process, but the cause is unknown. The features of idiopathic hypothyroidism resemble those found in chronic autoimmune thyroiditis (Hashimoto's disease). The plasma of patients with idiopathic hypothyroidism often contains thyroid antibodies, although the titer is not usually as high as in chronic autoimmune thyroiditis.[30] Secondly, abnormalities of intrathyroidal iodide metabolism, such as rapid iodide turnover and defective iodide organification, are found that are similar to those present in chronic autoimmune thyroiditis.[30] Finally, there are pathologic similarities between the two disorders, although the masses of thyroid tissue differ greatly, with chronic autoimmune thyroiditis being characterized by thyroid enlargement. These similarities have led many to conclude that these two diseases are closely related etiologically. Idiopathic hypothyroidism may be the end stage of an autoimmune process in which earlier thyroid enlargement was minimal or unrecognized.

CHRONIC AUTOIMMUNE THYROIDITIS (HASHIMOTO'S DISEASE)

Chronic autoimmune thyroiditis is a well-recognized cause of hypothyroidism. It may occur at any age, but it is most common in women in the third to sixth decades and is a common cause of hypothyroidism in children and adolescents. By definition thyroid enlargement is present. There are infiltrations with lymphocytes, plasma cells, and lymphoid germinal centers, as well as thyroid hyperplasia and varying degrees of fibrosis.[31] The thyroid enlargement may be either gradual or sudden. Clinical hypothyroidism is present in some patients; others are asymptomatic but have biochemical evidence of hypothyroidism such as elevated serum TSH concentrations. High titers of thyroid antibodies are found in most patients. Intrathyroidal defects in iodide metabolism are frequent, indicating that the disease process can result in quite specific defects in thyroid cell function.[30]

HYPOTHYROIDISM CAUSED BY ^{131}I THERAPY

Hypothyroidism occurring as a consequence of ^{131}I treatment for hyperthyroidism has become an important disorder and has received much study. Radiation damage caused by ^{131}I is limited to thyroid cells that concentrated the isotope. Therefore patients who develop hypothyroidism after ^{131}I therapy almost always have hyperthyroidism caused by Graves' disease. Hypothyroidism rarely occurs in patients given ^{131}I for uninodular or multinodular toxic goiter, since these patients have some suppressed thyroid tissue that does not concentrate the ^{131}I. Hypothyroidism can occur at any time after ^{131}I therapy. Its development soon after therapy is due to radiation-induced thyroid necrosis and is largely dose-related. Hypothyroidism within 1 year after therapy occurs in 4%–40% of patients given ^{131}I.[32-35] Hypothyroidism appearing 1 year or more after ^{131}I therapy occurs at a rate of 1%–3% per year, and current evidence indicates that new cases continue to appear indefinitely. Late hypothyroidism is not dependent on the initial ^{131}I dose, since new cases appear at similar rates in patients in whom the initial ^{131}I doses were small.[35] The continuing development of hypothyroidism after ^{131}I therapy reflects abnormal replication of ^{131}I-damaged thyroid cells, although until that time they function normally.

POSTOPERATIVE HYPOTHYROIDISM

Hypothyroidism may follow total or subtotal thyroidectomy. In the former procedure, which is usually done for the treatment of thyroid carcinoma, its occurrence is expected. Subtotal thyroidectomy, usually for the treatment of Graves' disease but occasionally to remove large multinodular goiters, is much more commonly performed. The reported incidences of hypothyroidism after subtotal thyroidectomy for Graves' disease vary from 5% to 30% in different reports,[32,34,36] but in many of these the duration of follow-up has been limited. One important factor is the size of the thyroid remnant. As is the case with ^{131}I therapy, new cases of postoperative hypothyroidism continue to occur indefinitely at the rate of 1%–2% per year.[34] This may reflect the natural history of Graves' disease rather than a late effect of surgery per se.[37]

TRANSIENT HYPOTHYROIDISM

Transient hypothyroidism may occur in patients after ^{131}I therapy, subtotal thyroidectomy for Graves' disease, or removal of an antonomously functioning thyroid adenoma.[38] It usually appears several weeks or months following the therapy and then gradually resolves as prior pituitary suppression disappears and the thyroid remnant enlarges. Subacute thyroiditis is also a cause of transient hypothyroidism, in which it develops after the acute inflammatory process subsides. The period of hypothyroidism may last several weeks or months, but full recovery almost always occurs.[39]

THYROID DYSGENESIS (SPORADIC NONGOITROUS CRETINISM)

Developmental defects of the thyroid gland are major causes of hypothyroidism occurring in the first months or years of life. Careful radioisotope studies have demonstrated that most patients have some thyroid tissue and that complete thyroid agenesis is rare. The thyroid tissue may be located in the middle anywhere from the base of the tongue to below the thyroid cartilage, or in the normal location on one or both sides of the neck.[40] The cause of such abnormal thyroid development is unknown.

Hypothyroidism Caused by Thyroid Biosynthetic Defects

Thyroid hormone biosynthesis and secretion are multistep processes that are to a large extent dependent on the TSH responsiveness of thyroid tissue. Genetically determined defects in many of these steps have been described. Most of these disorders are inherited as autosomal recessive traits. In the homozygote the thyroid deficiency leads to thyroid enlargement. This may be minimal early in life but may become marked later in childhood. In presumed heterozygotes the defect is usually mild, and only a slight degree of thyroid enlargement results. Specific defects thus far identified in such patients include abnormalities in iodide concentration, iodide organification, thyroglobulin biosynthesis, and iodotyrosine dehalogenase activity, as well as thyroidal insensitivity of thyrotropin.

Dietary iodide deficiency results in inadequate thyroid hormone production, despite the presence of intrinsically normal thyroid tissue. The occurrence of hypothyroidism (endemic cretinism) in regions where goiter caused by iodide deficiency is endemic is well known. The residents of such regions have high rates of thyroid enlargement, although the incidence varies widely in such populations; even greater are the incidences of abnormalities in thyroid iodide metabolism and secretion and elevated serum TSH concentrations. While the degree of iodide deficiency is undoubtedly the major determinant of the frequency of these findings, other variables such as diet, genetic factors, and water pollution may play a role in some endemic goiter areas.

Several inorganic and organic compounds, both naturally occurring and synthetic, have antithyroid actions. Since these compounds all inhibit thyroid hormone formation, usually by inhibiting iodide transport and organification, their administration can result in hypothyroidism with goiter. Widely used agents that may cause hypothyroidism and goiter are propylthiouracil, methimazole, iodide, and lithium carbonate. Many other drugs, chemicals, and constitutents of natural foodstuffs have antithyroid effects. These include thiocyanate, perchlorate, nitroprusside, sulfonamides, sulfonylureas, ethionamide, aminoglutethimide, resorcinol, and goitrin (found in various plants of the Brassicae family). These will not be further discussed, as their clinical significance is minimal or doubtful. Propylthiouracil and methimazole have well-recognized antithyroid effects, and hypothyroidism can result from their use in the therapy of hyperthyroidism. This may be manifested by the development of clinical manifestations of hypothyroidism and/or an enlarging thyroid gland. Iodide not only has antithyroid actions in patients with hyperthyroidism but also has recently been shown to have a slight transient antithyroid effect in normal subjects as well.[41] Goiter and hypothyroidism occurring during iodide administration have been recognized for some time.[42] They may be caused by inorganic iodide used alone or in proprietary expectorants and similar medications, or they may be caused by organic iodide compounds such as some drugs and radiographic contrast media. Iodide goiter and hypothyroidism seem to occur only in patients who have underlying thyroid disease, such as chronic autoimmune thyroiditis, or in patients treated with ^{131}I or surgical therapy for hyperthyroidism.[43] Maternal iodide ingestion can result in goiter and hypothyroidism in the fetus, and it appears that the fetal thyroid is more sensitive to the antithyroid effect of iodide. Lithium carbonate is perhaps the most commonly used "nonthyroid" drug that has an antithyroid action. In one survey of a large group of patients receiving lithium, 30 percent had some elevation of serum TSH concentrations. Clinical hypothyroidism with subnormal serum T4 concentrations was much less frequent.[44] As is the case with inorganic iodide, preexisting thyroid damage may increase susceptibility to lithium-induced hypothyroidism. The mechanism of the antithyroid action of lithium is not entirely clear; its major in vivo effect appears to be inhibition of thyroid hormone release.

Hypothyrotropic Hypothyroidism

Thyrotropin (SH) deficiency, either as the result of pituitary disease per se or deficiency of thyrotropin releasing hormone (TRH), is much less common than primary or thyroidal hypothyroidism. TSH deficiency may occur as a result of any type of pituitary disease; in most instances in adults it results from either functioning (growth hormone or prolactin secreting) or nonfunctioning pituitary adenomas.[45] If it is not present initially in such patients, TSH deficiency may result from surgical therapy or, less commonly, radiation therapy of such tumors. Other causes of TSH deficiency include postpartum pituitary necrosis (Sheehan's syndrome), pituitary cyst, craniopharyngioma, carotid aneurysm, trauma, hemochromatosis, and infiltrative processes such as tuberculosis and histiocytosis (Hand-Schüller-Christian disease). In other instances no cause is apparent; autoimmune mechanisms have been postulated but not established. In all of these situations TSH deficiency may occur in association with other tropic hormone deficiencies or as an isolated abnormality.

There is now strong circumstantial evidence that TRH deficiency can result in hypothyroidism, although secretion of TRH from the hypothalamus cannot be directly assessed. The basis for this diagnosis is the finding of low serum TSH concentrations that increase following the administration of TRH.[46] As with TSH deficiency, TRH deficiency may be isolated or may coexist with other tropic hormone deficiencies. The findings listed above may occur in patients with or without evident hypothalamic disease. Hypothalmic hypothyroidism has been described in a substantial portion of children previously considered to have idiopathic hypopituitarism, and it is likely that this disorder is frequently of hypothalamic origin.[47]

Hypothyroidism Caused by Peripheral Resistance to Thyroid Hormones

A few patients have been reported in whom there was partial peripheral resistance to thyroid hormone.[48-50] These patients were clinically euthyroid, with elevated serum thyroid hormone levels and thyroid enlargement; exogenous thyroid hormone had little effect. Several patients had physical findings (such as deafness and stippled epiphyses) indicative of hypothyroidism in their past; others were entirely normal or had thyroid enlargement. Complete end-organ resistance to thyroid hormones would no doubt result in severe infantile hypothyroidism no matter how much thyroid hormone could be produced. The nature of the defect or defects in thyroid hormone responsiveness in these patients is unknown.

BIOCHEMICAL MANIFESTATIONS AND LABORATORY DIAGNOSIS

Decreased production of thyroxine (T4) and triiodothyronine (T3) is the physiologic abnormality common to all forms of hypothyroidism. The best readily measurable hallmark of hypothyroidism is a decreased serum total T4 concentration, as measured by competitive protein binding analysis (T4-D) or radioimmunoassay (T4-RIA). Decreased serum free T4 concentrations are also present. Serum thyroxine binding globulin (TBG) and thyroxine binding prealbumin (TBPA) capacities are normal. Serum T3 resin uptake tests indicate that there is an increased number of unoccupied binding sites; hence low values for tests such as the free thyroxine index and adjusted thyroxine index are found. It is important to recognize that the serum T4 concentration need not be definitely subnormal in the presence of significant hypothyroidism. Conversely, a low serum T4 concentration does not always reflect the presence of hypothyroidism. Some patients with thyroid damage have low serum T4 concentrations, but they are not hypothyroid, and serum T3 and TSH concentrations are normal.[51] Administration of triiodothyronine to normal patients, as well as to hypothyroid patients, is associated with a low serum T4 concentration. The serum T4 concentration also may be reduced as a result of decreased production or loss of TBG, or it may be reduced by agents such as salicylate that competitively inhibit the T4–TBG interaction. In the latter instances T3 resin tests indicate a decrease in unoccupied T4 binding sites; the serum free T4 concentration and tests indirectly reflecting it are normal.

Since most serum T3 is produced by extrathyroidal deiodination of T4, the serum T3 concentration is usually low in patients with hypothyroidism. However, a low serum T3 concentration is neither as sensitive nor as specific an indicator of hypothyroidism as is a low serum T4 level. About 30 percent of hypothyroid patients with low serum T4 concentrations have normal serum T3 concentrations.[52] This finding reflects maintenance of a more nearly normal thyroidal T3 secretion than T4 secretion as a consequence of excessive TSH stimulation of the thyroid gland. Also, serum T3 concentrations are subnormal

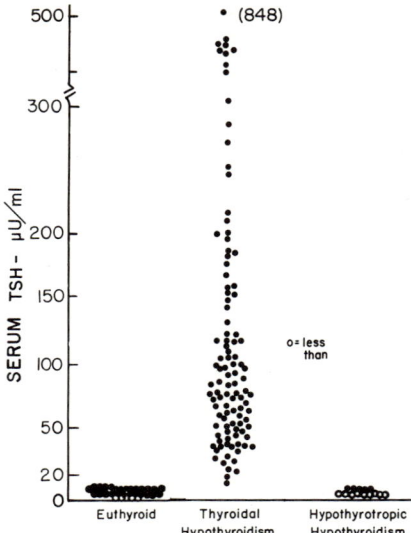

Fig. 2–2. Serum TSH concentrations in normal subjects and patients with thyroidal hypothyroidism and hypothyrotropic hypothyroidism.

in patients with many other illnesses who appear euthyroid and have normal serum T4 and TSH concentrations.[53,54] These include chronic cardiac, renal, hepatic, and respiratory insufficiency, malnutrition, and anorexia nervosa. The low serum T3 concentrations in these situations reflect decreased extrathyroidal conversion of T4 to T3. Why T4-to-T3 conversion is impaired in these situations is not known, nor are the physiologic consequences of this abnormality known.

Measurements of serum TSH concentrations by radioimmunoassay are very useful for diagnosis of thyroidal hypothyroidism and differentiation of thyroidal from hypothyrotropic hypothyroidism. Results of serum TSH determinations in normal subjects and patients with thyroidal hypothyroidism and hypothyrotropic hypothyroidism are shown in Figure 2–2. In virtually all patients with symptomatic thyroidal hypothyroidism, serum TSH concentrations are unequivocally elevated. Serum TSH concentrations also are often elevated in patients with chronic autoimmune thyroiditis and in patients who have had subtotal thyroidectomy or ^{131}I therapy, even though they are clinically euthyroid and their serum T4 and T3 concentrations are within the normal range.[55-57] Such a finding does not indicate imminent symptomatic hypothyroidism. In contrast, serum TSH concentrations are normal or undetectable in most patients with pituitary or hypothalmic hypothyroidism. Characteristically, serum TSH concentrations fail to rise following TRH administration in patients with pituitary hypothyroidism. Many euthyroid patients with pituitary disease also have a subnormal TSH response to TRH, i.e., TSH reserve is limited.[45] Substantial (but sometimes delayed) increases are characteristic of hypothalamic hypothyroidism,[46] but similar responses occur in some patients with overt pituitary disease.[45] In patients with thyroidal hypothyroidism the TSH response to TRH is greater than normal. Figure 2–3 shows the characteristic patterns of serum TSH response after TRH administration in patients with thyroidal, pituitary, and hypothalamic hypothyroidism.

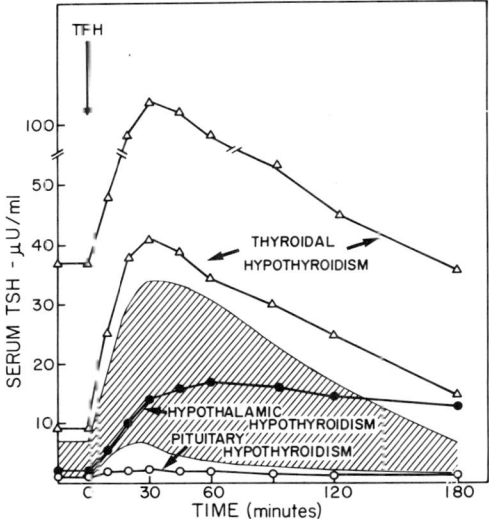

Fig. 2–3. Typical serum TSH responses to TRH in patients with different types of hypothyroidism. The diagonal lines indicate the range of TSH responses to TRH in normal subjects.

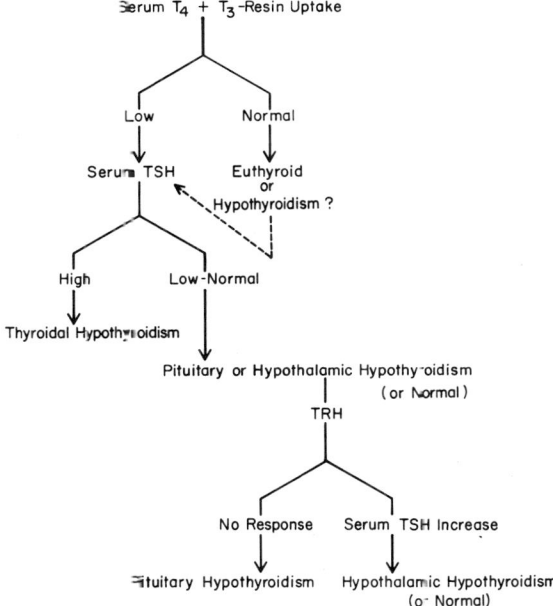

Fig. 2–4. Outline for the laboratory evaluation of patients suspected of having hypothyroidism.

An outline for the evaluation of a patient with clinically suspected hypothyroidism, based largely on simple tests that are widely available, is shown in Figure 2–4. These procedures should confirm the diagnosis of hypothyroidism and establish its origin (but not its cause) in most patients.

Other tests of thyroid function have been described, but they are rarely needed. The most widely used in the past was estimation of thyroidal ^{131}I uptake. Characteristically this is reduced in patients with hypothyroidism. The value of thyroidal ^{131}I uptake tests has declined because increased dietary iodide has resulted in lower values for percentage ^{131}I uptake in normal individuals. Therefore, recognition of subnormal uptake is very difficult. Furthermore, additional iodide intake (such as from drugs or contrast media) reduces ^{131}I uptake to very low levels in normal individuals. Tests for antithyroid antibodies may suggest the cause of thyroid enlargement or hypothyroidism, but they do not provide information concerning thyroid secretion.

Hypothyroidism is accompanied by numerous biochemical changes that reflect decreased tissue actions of thyroid hormones. The basal metabolic rate is reduced. The Achilles reflex half-relaxation time is prolonged.[10] Serum concentrations of various enzymes, cholesterol, triglycerides, and carotene are frequently elevated. All of these findings, when encountered unexpectedly, may suggest the presence of hypothyroidism. Such procedures should never be used to confirm the diagnosis, since specific and sensitive direct measurements of thyroid and pituitary secretion are available.

THERAPY OF HYPOTHYROIDISM

The general principle is simple: restore and maintain the euthyroid state. The initial dose of thyroid hormone should be small, since rapid restoration of normal metabolic activity occasionally precipitates angina pectoris, cardiac arrhythmias, or cardiac failure. Thus most older patients should be given one-third to one-half the expected replacement dose. When there is a history of cardiac disease, more caution is warranted. The replacement dosage should not be increased until the full effects of a given dose are achieved. The time required for this varies, but it is several weeks for T3 and longer (perhaps 4–6 weeks) for T4. In younger patients less caution is necessary. The rate of response depends on the dose and the preparation used. With T4 there may be some subjective improvement in the first week or so. An increase in pulse rate, the appearance of diuresis, and decreases in serum TSH, cholesterol, and creatinine phosphokinase concentrations are usually the first objective changes noted, occuring in 1–2 weeks. With moderate but incomplete replacement doses, most symptoms improve or disappear in 1–2 months. Certain abnormalities, such as anemia and abnormal cortisol and growth hormone secretory patterns, may not return to normal for many months.[58]

Estimation of the adequacy of therapy may be based on the disappearance of symptoms and signs, on restoration of normal serum TSH concentrations (in patients with thyroidal hypothyroidism), or on a combination of these. Clinical response alone usually is sufficient. Serum T4 concentrations during therapy depend on the type of hormone used. Since the range of serum T4 concentrations in normal subjects is wide and the normal concentration for any individual is not known, the restoration of any normal serum T4 concentration may not be appropriate. An elevated serum TSH concentration is good evidence that therapy is inadequate. However, this measurement cannot be used to recognize overtreatment, since some normal individuals have barely detectable or undetectable

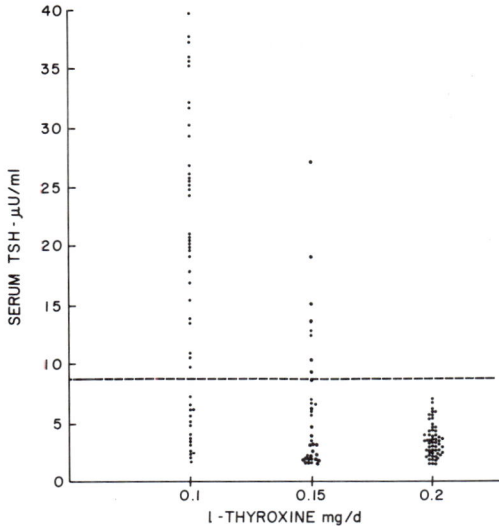

Fig. 2–5. Serum TSH concentrations in hypothyroid patients treated chronically with thyroxine. The results indicate that 0.15 mg daily provides adequate replacement in most (but not all) of such patients. The dashed line indicates the upper limit of normal.

serum TSH concentrations (Fig. 2–2). The major difficulty, however, is the frequency with which therapy is discontinued by patients, no matter how often they are informed that the need is lifelong.

A number of preparations are available for the treatment of hypothyroidism. These include synthetic L-thyroxine, synthetic L-triiodothyronine, combinations of the two, and desiccated thyroid and thryoglobulin. In appropriate doses, all provide complete symptomatic relief. Serum TSH concentrations in adult patients with previously proven thyroidal hypothyroidism treated chronically with various doses of T4 are shown in Figure 2–5. Most patients have normal serum TSH concentrations while receiving 0.15–0.2 mg of T4 daily. Equivalent doses of desiccated thyroid are 90–120 mg daily, and those of T3 are 50–75 μg daily. The choice of the preparation to be used is perhaps less important than selection of the proper dosage. Both theoretic and practical reasons make L-thyroxine the preparation of choice. The rise in both serum T4 and T3 concentrations after initiation of therapy is gradual, and appropriate doses result in normal serum concentrations of both.[52] Furthermore, in chronically treated patients a single daily dose of T4 does not produce fluctuations of serum T4, T3, or TSH concentrations.[59] Thus T4 therapy reproduces normal physiology. In contrast, serum T3 concentrations fluctuate markedly after single doses of T3 alone or doses of T4 and T3 combined,[59] often reaching values two to four times normal several hours after T3 administration. While it is difficult to demonstrate changing tissue effects of these varying serum T3 concentrations, some patients may have transient subjective symptoms of thyroid hormone excess after T3 administration. Furthermore, neither serum T3 nor serum T4 determinations are useful in assessing the adequacy of therapy, since serum T3 concentrations fluctuate so much following T3 administration and serum T4 concentrations are low normal to low no matter how much or how little therapeutic benefit has been obtained.

REFERENCES

1. Wantanakunakorn C, Hodges RH, Evans TC: Myxedema: A study of 400 cases. Arch Intern Med 116:183, 1965
2. Wayne EJ: Clinical and metabolic studies in thyroid disease. Br Med J 1:1, 78, 1960
3. Oddie TH, Boyd CM, Fisher DA, et al: Incidence of signs and symptoms in thyroid disease. Med J Aust 2:981, 1972
4. De Groot LJ, Stanbury JB: The Thyroid and Its Diseases (ed 4). New York, John Wiley, 1975, pp. 440–441
5. Billewicz WZ, Chapman RS, Crooks J, et al: Statistical methods applied to the diagnosis of hypothyroidism. Q J Med 38:255, 1969
6. Li MC, Rall JE, MacLean JP, et al: Thyroid function following hypophysectomy in man. J Clin Endocrinol Metab 15:1228, 1955
7. Sensenbach W, Madison L, Eisenberg S, et al: The cerebral circulation and metabolism in hyperthyroidism and myxedema. J Clin Invest 33:1434, 1954
8. Blum M: Myxedema coma. Am J Med Sci 264:432, 1972
9. Sanders V: Neurologic manifestations of myxedema. N Engl J Med 266:547, 599, 1962
10. Shafer RB, Nuttall FQ: Achilles reflex in thyroid disorders: A 10 year clinical evaluation. Am J Med Sci 264:313, 1972
11. Nickel SN, Frame B, Bebin J, et al: Myxedema neuropathy and myopathy. Neurology 11:125–137, 1961
12. Bland JH, Frymoyer JW: Rheumatic syndromes of myxedema. N Engl J Med 282:1171, 1970
13. Buccino RA, Spann JF Jr, Pool PE, et al: Influence of the thyroid state on the intrinsic contractile properties and the energy stores of the myocardium. J Clin Invest 46:1669, 1967
14. Graetinger JS, Meunster JJ, Checchia CS, et al: A correlation of clinical and hemodynamic studies in patients with hypothyroidism. J Clin Invest 37:502, 1958
15. Fleisher GA, McConahey WM, Pankow M: Serum creatine kinase, lactic dehydrogenase and glutamic-oxalacetic transaminase in thyroid diseases and pregnancy. Mayo Clin Proc 40:300, 1965
16. Vanhaelst L, Neve P, Chailly P, et al: Coronary-artery disease in hypothyroidism. Lancet 2:800, 1967
17. Steinberg AD: Myxedema and coronary artery disease — A comparative autopsy study. Ann Intern Med 68:338, 1968
18. Wilson WR, Bedell GN: The pulmonary abnormalities in myxedema. J Clin Invest 39:42, 1960
19. Tudhope GD, Wilson GM: Deficiency of vitamin B_{12} in hypothyroidism. Lancet 1:703, 1962
20. Tulloch BR, Lewis B, Fraser TR: Triglyceride metabolism in thyroid disease. Lancet 1:391, 1973
21. Das KC, Mukherjee M, Sarkar TK, et al: Erythropoiesis and erythropoietin in hypo- and hyperthyroidism. J Clin Endocrinol Metab 40:211, 1975
22. Peterson RE: The influence of the thyroid on adrenal cortical function. J Clin Invest 37:736, 1958
23. Kaplan NM: Methopyrapone test in primary hypothyroidism. J Clin Endocrinol Metab 25:146, 1965
24. Havard CWH, Saldanha VF, Bird R, et al: Adrenal function in hypothyroidism. Br Med J 1:337, 1970
25. Akande EO: Plasma concentration of gonadotropins, oestrogen and progesterone in hypothyroid women. Br J Obstet Gynecol 82:552, 1975
26. MacGillirray MH, Aceto T Jr, Frohman LA: Plasma growth hormone responses and growth retardation of hypothyroidism. Am J Dis Child 115:273, 1968
27. Snyder PJ, Jacobs LS, Utiger RD, et al: Thyroid hormone inhibition of prolactin response to thyrotropin releasing hormone. J Clin Invest 52:2324, 1973
28. Boroditsky RS, Faiman C: Galactorrhea-amenorrhea due to primary hypothyroidism. Am J Obstet Gynecol 116:661, 1973
29. Sclere G: The thyroid in myxedema. J Pathol Bacteriol 85: 263, 1963
30. Buchanan WN, Harden RM: Primary hypothyroidism and Hashimoto's thyroiditis. Arch Intern Med 115:411, 1965
31. Woolner LB, McConahey WM, Beahrs OH: Struma lymphomatosa (Hashimoto's thyroiditis) and related thyroid disorders. J Clin Endocrinol Metab 19:53, 1959
32. Green M, Wilson GM: Thyrotoxicosis treated by surgery or iodine[131], with special reference as development of hypothyroidism. Br Med J 1:1005, 1964
33. Dunn JT, Chapman EM: Rising incidence of hypothyroidism after radioactive-iodine therapy in thyrotoxicosis. N Engl J Med 271:1037, 1964
34. Nofal MM, Bierwaltes WH: Treatment of hyperthyroidism with sodium iodide-I[131]. JAMA 197:605, 1966
35. Glennon JA, Gordon ES, Sawin, CT: Hypothyroidism after low-dose ^{131}I treatment of hyperthyroidism. Ann Intern Med 76:721, 1972
36. Hershman JM: The treatment of hyperthyroidism. Ann Intern Med 64:1306, 1966
37. Wood LC, Peterson M, Ingbar SH: Delayed

hypothyroidism following antithyroid therapy in Graves' disease. Clin Res 20:525, 1972
38. Toft AD, Seth J, Hunter WM, et al: Plasma-thyrotrophin and serum-thyroxine in patients becoming hypothyroid in the early months after iodine[131]. Lancet 1:704, 1974
39. Gordin A, Lamberg BA: Serum thyrotrophin response to thyrotrophin releasing hormone and the concentration of free thyroxine in subacute thyroiditis. Acta Endocrinol (Kbh) 74:111, 1973
40. Strickland AL, Macfie JA, Van Wyk JJ, et al: Ectopic thyroid glands simulating thyroglossal duct cysts. JAMA 208:307, 1969
41. Vagenakis AG, Downs P, Braverman LE, et al: Control of thyroid hormone secretion in normal subjects receiving iodides. J Clin Invest 52:528, 1973
42. Wolff J: Iodide goiter and the pharmacologic effects of excess iodide. Am J Med 47:101, 1969
43. Braverman LE, Woeber KA, Ingbar SH: Induction of myxedema by iodide in patients euthyroid after radioiodine or surgical treatment of diffuse toxic goiter. N Engl J Med 281:816, 1969
44. Emerson CH, Dyson WL, Utiger RD: Serum thyrotropin and thyroxine concentrations in patients receiving lithium carbonate. J Clin Endocrinol Metab 36:338, 1973
45. Snyder PJ, Jacobs LS, Rabello MM, et al: diagnostic value of thyrotrophin-releasing hormone in pituitary and hypothalamic diseases: Assessment of thyrotrophin and prolactin secretion in 100 patients. Ann Intern Med 81:751, 1974
46. Snyder PJ, Utiger RD: Repetitive administration of thyrotropin-releasing hormone results in small elevations of serum thyroid hormones and in marked inhibition of thyrotropin response. J Clin Invest 52:2305, 1973
47. Kaplan SL, Grumbach MM, Friesen HG, et al: Thyrotropin-releasing factor (TRF) effect on secretion of human pituitary prolactin and thyrotropin in children and in idiopathic hypopituitary dwarfism: Further evidence for hypophysiotropic hormone deficiencies. J Clin Endocrinol Metab 35:825, 1972
48. Refetoff S, De Groot LJ, Benard B, et al: Studies of a sibship with apparent hereditary resistance to the intracellular action of thyroid hormone. Metabolism 21:723, 1972
49. Bode HH, Danon M, Weintraub BD, et al: Partial target organ resistance to thyroid hormone. J Clin Invest 52:776, 1973
50. Lamberg BA: Congenital euthyroid goitre and partial peripheral resistance to thyroid hormones Lancet 1:854, 1973
51. Sterling K, Brenner MA, Newman ES, et al: The significance of triiodothyronine (T3) in maintenance of euthyroid status after treatment of hyperthyroidism. J Clin Endocrinol Metab 33:729 1971
52. Utiger RD: Serum triiodothyronine in man. Ann Rev Med 25:289, 1974
53. Carter JN, Eastman, CJ, Corcoran JM, et al: Effect of severe, chronic illness on thyroid function. Lancet 2:971, 1974
54. Bermudez F, Surks MI, Oppenheimer JH: High incidence of decreased serum triiodothyronine concentrations in patients with non-thyroidal disease. J Clin Endocrinol Metab 41:27, 1975
55. Mayberry WE, Gharib H, Bilstad JM et al: Radioimmunoassay for human thyrotrophin Ann Intern Med 74:471, 1971
56. Hedley AJ, Hall R, Amos J, et al: Serum-thyrotropin levels after subtotal thyroidectomy for Graves' disease. Lancet 1:455, 1971
57. Tunbridge WMG, Harsoulis P, Goolden AWG: Thyroid function in patients treated with radioactive iodine for thyrotoxicosis. Br Med J 2:89, 1974
58. Ridgway, EC, McCammon JA, Benotti J, et al: Acute metabolic responses in myxedema to large doses of intravenous L-thyroxine. Ann Intern Med 77:549, 1972
59. Saberi M, Utiger RD: Serum thyroid hormone and thyrotropin concentrations during thyroxine and triiodothyronine therapy. J Clin Endocrinol Metab 39:923, 1974

Stephen Richardson
and Charles S. Hollander

3
T3 Toxicosis and Its Clinical Variants: A Reappraisal

It has been 25 years since the discovery of triiodothyronine (T3) and documentation of its existence in the blood. In this chapter we will describe the development of accurate and sensitive radioimmunoassay procedures for the measurement of T3 in blood, demonstrate how these have led to a fuller appreciation of the physiologic significance of T3, and define those aspects of its role in human physiology that remain to be clarified. In the process we will delineate the syndrome of T3 toxicosis and its clinical variants, since these instances of hyperthyroidism, on the basis of excessive production of T3 with normal thyroxine (T4) levels, are probably the most dramatic clinical documentation of a significant role for T3 in human physiology.

BACKGROUND

In 1952 Gross and Pitt-Rivers[1] carefully examined the circulating thyroid hormones in the plasma of 6 patients with hyperthyroidism after the administration of therapeutic doses of radioactive iodine. Although their methodology (which involved chemical extraction, paper chromatography, and a modified Kieselguhr column) was crude by current standards, they were able to extract a substance previously referred to only as unknown I from human serum and to demonstrate convincingly that this compound was 3,5,3'-L-triiodothyronine or T3. This finding, which was soon corroborated by Roche, Lissitsky, and Michel[2] and subsequently by many others, opened a new era in thyroidology.

It soon became apparent from experimental studies in animals and later clinical observations in man that his new congener of thyroid hormone was more potent metabolically than was thyroxine. However, full appreciation of its considerable physiologic and biologic significance came only after the development of reliable, sensitive, and accurate methods for its measurement. To comprehend why this was such a difficult task, it is necessary to recall that the total measurable organic iodine is only of the order of $9\mu g/dl$, that T3 and T4 closely resemble each other, and that the concentration of T3 is less than 2 percent that of T4, which accounts for 85–90 percent of the organic iodine-containing compounds in the blood. Thus it is perhaps understandable that it has taken almost 20 years to develop accurate measurements of T3 in serum. A logical corollary of these physiologic findings would be that hyperthyroidism could develop on the basis of an elevated serum T3 level in the presence of a normal serum T4 level. A few cases where this situation apparently existed were described quite early after the discovery of T3. However, these were really presumptive, as no reliable method of precisely measuring serum T3 levels had been formulated.

Radiochromatography was the method initially used by most workers to measure T3 levels, but in 1957 MacLagan et al.[3] described a chromatographic process and a chemical quantitation of iodine not involving radioiodine administration to the subjects studied. They found T3 present in both normal and thyrotoxic subjects, and it was much more easily detected in the latter group. Some of their results indicated an excess of T3 but not T4 in the serum of thyrotoxic patients, and they suggested the importance of T3 in hyperthyroidism.

Patients with excess T3 in the serum were also reported by other authors. For example, in 1959 Rupp et al.[4] described a 23-year-old woman with a large nontoxic goiter of 9 years duration with a normal PBI and an elevated ^{131}I iodoprotein level suggestive of a raised serum T3 concentration. Werner et al.[5] described a 16-year-old girl who also had a large nontoxic goiter. T3 was the main iodine-containing compound in her serum, as well as in one of the lobes of the thyroid. A patient with metastatic carcinoma of the thyroid who had a high serum T3:T4 ratio was reported by Mack et al.[6] However, the suggestion that an elevated T3 might be responsible for hyperthyroidism was first made by Rupp and Paschkis[7] in 1961. They described a 19-year-old girl who had clinical evidence of Graves' disease. Her PBI was 6.5 µg/dl, and radiochromatographic studies indicated an elevated serum T3 level. The same method was used by Shimaoka[8] in 1963 to measure an elevated T3 in a thyrotoxic patient with a solitary thyroid adenoma. In 1964 Czerniak and Chaitchik[9] reported a series of 10 patients with hyperthyroidism, all of whom had elevated T3 levels.

In none of these cases could the diagnosis of T3 toxicosis be stated unequivocally, for in addition to the difficulty of accurately measuring T3, the free thyroxine and thyroxine binding capacity of thyroid binding proteins had not been determined. It is worthwhile to mention at this point that very little naturally occurring thyroxine is in the free form (approximately 0.04 percent), whereas the vast majority is bound to thyroxine binding globulin (TBG) or thyroxine binding albumin and prealbumin (TBPA). T3 has greater potency than T4 and also a shorter half-life, which has been ascribed to its weaker protein binding. This means that T3 has a greater volume of distribution than T4 and that a greater (but still small) proportion of T3 is in the free form (0.3 percent). These physiologic observations form the basis for the suggestion that hyperthyroidism may be caused by an elevated T3 without a raised PBI; they also help explain why T3 is not only more active metabolically than T4 but also more rapid in action.

The first well-documented case of T3 toxicosis was reported in 1968 by Hollander,[10] who used a sophisticated gas-liquid chromatographic (GLC) method to measure T3. The patient was a 62-year-old man with clinical evidence of hyperthyroidism. His BMR was +40 percent, PBI was 5.6 and 6.1 µg/dl (normal 4–8 µg/dl), and ^{131}I uptake was 69 percent at 24 hr. He had a normal T4, but elevated T3, as measured using the GLC method. His T4 secretion rate was normal, but his T3 secretion rate was elevated. This patient later developed severe clinical disease with congestive heart failure. He eventually underwent partial thyroidectomy and made a good recovery, with return of T3 levels to normal. Hollander et al. subsequently described several other cases in which they used the same methodology.[11]

At about the same time Nauman et al.[12] and later Sterling et al.[13] described a competitive protein binding method for T3 assay. Sterling described a case of Graves' disease and a patient with a toxic nodular goiter with elevated T3 levels and normal T4 levels; he recorded results form 23 similar patients. The competitive binding protein method requires extraction of thyroid hormones from serum, separation of T3 from T4, elution of the separated T3, and measurement of the T3 by a competitive protein binding technique. It is now generally agreed that this method overestimates the true level of T3 because of contamination of chromatographically pure T3 by T4 and because of in vitro conversion of T4 to T3. These problems may cause overestimation of the true level of T3 by as much as 50–100%.

Gas-liquid chromatography also proved to be a time-consuming and difficult procedure. It necessitated extraction of T3 from serum using a cation-exchange resin column preparation of a stable and volatile T3 derivative and its purification with further ion resin exchange procedures and finally separation and quantitation by gas chromatography. Again, in vitro conversion of T4 to T3 was a problem. To overcome this, T4 was added to the system to determine variations in measured T3, and an empirically determined conversion factor was used to convert for the T4-to-T3 conversion. With this significant modification the method was both accurate and reproducible, but it was too cumbersome for routine use.

RADIOIMMUNOASSAY METHODS

As we have seen, early investigators resorted to radiochromatographic, gas-liquid chromatographic, and competitive binding assay procedures in their initial attempts to measure T3. T3 and T4 radioimmunoassay techniques have subsequently been developed and are now very accurate and relatively easy to perform. It is surprising that such a development for thyroid hormones has lagged 10 years behind similar techniques used for other hormones. This was probably largely because of initial doubt that antibodies with the requisite sensitivity and affinity could effectively be raised against a molecule as small as T3. By the late 1960s and early 1970s it became apparent that this technical problem could be largely circumvented by conjugating the antigen with a haptene such as albumin, globulin, poly-L-lysine, or the like. Brown et al.[14] were first to demonstrate the feasibility of raising such an antibody to T3. Our group developed a rapid and sensitive radioimmunoassay for T3 in serum, and similar procedures have been reported by others. The procedure actually permits the simultaneous measurement of T4, but we will concentrate on the T3 assay exclusively. Three basic steps analogous to those of other immunoassays are performed: (1) immunization of rabbits with a T3-haptene-linked immunogen and harvest of specific antibodies to T3, (2) addition of isotopically labeled tracer levels of T3 to standards or to the unknown and unlabeled T3, and (3) separation of T3 that is bound to the antibody from free (i.e., unbound) hormone.

The details of the assay have been published previously,[15] but several features are perhaps worthy of mention:

1. To perform the assay in unextracted serum, the binding of T3 to serum proteins must be inhibited by a suitable blocking agent. In our initial studies we utilized tetrachlorthyronine for this purpose, while other workers used Dilantin[16] and salicylates.[17] In subsequent studies we have resorted to 8-anilino-1-naphthalene sulfonic acid (ANS) to achieve the same end,[18] and Chopra et al.[19] have also employed ANS in this

manner. Other workers have obtained comparable results by separating T3 from plasma proteins using extraction on a Sephadex G-25 column[20] or methanol.[21]
2. By using dextran-coated charcoal to achieve a rapid separation of the bound and free isotope moieties and by performing the incubation for 90 min at 37°C, it is possible to complete the entire procedure in 3–4 hr.
3. Our T3 antiserum showed a cross-reaction to T4 of less than 1:5000, which is of considerable importance in view of the very low levels of T3 relative to that of T4.

Although there was initially considerable controversy over the true levels of circulating T3, it is now generally accepted that the mean T3 in normal adults is somewhere between 100 and 160 ng/dl.[22]

CLINICAL PICTURE OF T3 TOXICOSIS

Subsequent to the development of an accurate, rapid, and sensitive radioimmunoassay we published a study of 40 patients with T3 toxicosis.[23] The diagnosis was made on the basis of clinical evidence of hyperthyroidism with normal total T4 and free T4 levels and elevated T3 levels. Twenty-nine of the patients had typical Graves' disease, 8 patients had single autonomous thyroid nodules, and 3 patients had toxic multinodular goiters. Thirty-one of these patients were female, and their ages varied from 22 to 83 years. In the patients with Graves' disease the mean T3 level was 807 ng/dl (normal range 96–172 ng/dl); in those with solitary adenomata it was 525 ng/dl; and in the toxic multinodular goiter group it was 285 ng/dl. The mean percentage free T3 overall was 0.26 (normal 0.15–0.32), and the mean free T3 was 1.92 ng/dl (normal 0.1–0.5 ng/dl).

Carter et al.[24] recently reported 3 patients with T3 toxicosis and summarized data from 131 other patients from the world literature. They concluded that conventional hyperthyroidism and T3 toxicosis are generally similar but that the latter tends to be less severe and that the reported incidence of T3 toxicosis among thyrotoxic patients varies between 4 and 12.5 percent. The age of onset of T3 toxicosis is variable, and cases have been reported in young children[25] and in an 83-year-old woman, but the average age of onset is higher than in conventional thyrotoxicosis.[24]

As in our own series, T3 toxicosis can present in any of the common guises of conventional hyperthyroidism, i.e., Graves' disease, toxic multinodular goiter, and autonomous adenoma. T3 toxicosis has also been described in patients with disseminated follicular carcinoma of the thyroid[26] and Hashimoto's thyroiditis.[27] Moreover administration of iodide[28] and desiccated thyroid extract and imipramine[29] has also been incriminated in the provocation of T3 toxicosis. Often elevated T3 levels are responsible for those cases of borderline hyperthyroidism where the diagnosis is suspected but cannot be confirmed by conventional thyroid function studies. However, all degrees of thyrotoxicity have been noted in association with T3 toxicosis. For example, apathetic thyrotoxicosis due to T3 has been described,[30] and so has the "thyroid storm" syndrome.[31] A case of periodic paralysis in T3 toxicosis was reported from Japan.[32] Thus it would appear that there are no special features of thyrotoxicosis that are peculiar to or pathognomonic of either T3 toxicosis or conventional hyperthyroidism. There is little correlation between the level of total T3 and the degree of thyrotoxicosis, and the same is true of T4. However, a possible rough correlation between the degree of thyrotoxicosis and the free T3 concentration was suggested in our series of 40 patients.[23]

CLINICAL VARIANTS

T3 Toxicosis as a Premonitory Finding in Conventional Hyperthyroidism

Although we have thus far discussed the syndrome of T3 toxicosis and conventional hyperthyroidism as entirely separate entities, there are instances in which the distinction between the two becomes less clear. In 1971 Hollander et al.[33] described 4 clinically euthyroid patients with elevated T3 and normal T4 levels who within 5 weeks to 9 months went on to develop conventional thyrotoxicosis with clinical and biochemical evidence, including raised T3 levels. The diagnosis was difficult before obvious clinical evidence was available. One patient gave a history of nervous irritability for 7 months. Another patient with exophthalmos and pretibial myxedema had a normal T4 for 10 months in the presence of a raised T3. A third patient had a past history of drug treatment for hyperthyroidism before developing T3 toxicosis. Although the true incidence of transient T3 toxicosis is unknown, these findings do raise the possibility that T3 toxicosis may sometimes be a premonitory finding in conventional hyperthyroidism.

T3 Toxicosis in the Course of Drug Therapy

A 30-year-old man with conventional hyperthyroidism was controlled with drug therapy. When the dosage was lowered he developed T3 toxicosis, and when it was increased again he became clinically euthyroid once more, with a normal T4 level. This case, reported by our group,[34] illustrates that T3 toxicosis may develop during the course of suboptimal drug therapy; Bellabarba[35] has observed a similar phenomenon.

T3 Toxicosis as a Harbinger of Recurrence

We have already seen that T3 toxicosis may be the first premonitory finding in conventional hyperthyroidism. Our group was also first to suggest that T3 toxicosis may often be the harbinger of recurrence of thyroid overactivity.[36] In a group of 10 patients, elevation of T3 was the first biochemical abnormality to appear, and recurrence took place after intervals varying from 6 months to 30 years. In looking at a group of thyrotoxic patients, Marsden and McKerron[37] found that 18 of 46 patients had recurrent Graves' disease and that 2 of these patients developed T3 toxicosis. They also noted that the T3:T4 ratio was greater in recurrent cases than in new cases of Graves' disease; they suggested that T3 may play a more important role than T4 in the pathophysiology of recurrent Graves' disease.

T3 Toxicosis in the Presence of Iodine Deficiency

The association of iodine deficiency and T3 toxicosis has also been well described.[38] Whereas the incidence of T3 toxicosis in New York has been estimated to be about 4 percent of all hyperthyroid patients, workers in Santiago, Chile, a relatively iodine-deficient area, were surprised to find a large number of patients with obvious clinical hyperthyroidism but with normal protein-bound iodine (PBI) levels with elevated radioactive iodine uptake (56 patients out of 393 patients with clinical hyperthyroidism over the course of 2 years). We had the opportunity to study 12 of these 56 patients in detail. All patients had clinical hyperthyroidism, and 7 patients had eye signs. Radioactive iodine uptake was raised in 8 patients. In all 12 patients the serum PBI and total and free T4 levels were normal, T3 levels were raised (260–840 ng/dl; normal range 96–172 ng/dl), and serum TSH levels were below 0.25 μU/ml (normal range from undetectable or less than 0.25 μU/ml to 3.5 μU/ml). In 2 patients the urinary iodide output was studied and was found to be low (34 and 39 μg/24 hr; normal 50 μg/24 hr or more). The apparently great difference in the incidences of T3 toxicosis in New York and Santiago is striking and suggests that iodine deficiency affects the relative production of T3 and T4. Similar preferential secretion of T3 over T4 with iodine deficiency has also been demonstrated in animals[39,40] and would appear to be a logical adaptation of thyroid metabolism, in view of the fact that T3 has about four times the metabolic activity of T4 and requires 25 percent less iodide for its formation.

SOURCES OF T3 IN THE CIRCULATION

Thyroidal secretion of T3 was unequivocally documented by Taurog et al.[41] shortly following the discovery of T3 by Gross and Pitt-Rivers[1] in 1952. Gross[42] suggested that T3 was also derived from peripheral conversion of T4, but early attempts to document this produced conflicting results.[43,44] More recently it has been clearly demonstrated that a substantial proportion of circulating T3 is derived by this pathway, although its precise quantitative contribution remains controversial.

T4 undergoes a number of metabolic transformations in addition to the one that produces T3. One well-documented alternate pathway involves deamination of the side chain to give rise to tetraiodothyroacetic acid, or tetrac. Recently considerable attention has focused on an alternate monodeiodination pathway in which a single iodine is lost in the inner (alpha) carboxyl ring instead of the outer (beta) phenolic ring. Thus monodeiodination may give rise not only to T3 itself but also to a noncalorigenic congener of T3: reverse T3 (3,3′,5-triiodothyronine). Moreover, in the case of reverse T3 (rT3) peripheral conversion accounts for the large bulk of its production, with thyroidal secretion contributing only 2.5 percent of its production.[45] Therefore it might be anticipated that in T3 toxicosis rT3 levels might provide a hint concerning the source of the excessive T3 in the circulation. Griffiths et al.[46] has found normal rT3 levels in 16 patients with T3 toxicosis, and the range was similar to that found in a group of euthyroid patients with equivalent T4 values. This could be consistent with a thyroidal source for the T3. On the other hand, Herrmann et al.[47] and Wenzel and Meinhold[48] have observed low rT3 levels in these patients, suggesting that at least some cases of T3 toxicosis may be caused by an abnormality in the relative proportion of monodeiodination of the alpha and beta rings, viz., in periphheral conversion. A recent observation of considerable interest is that during caloric deprivation in euthyroid patients the T4 level remains normal, the T3 level falls, and the rT3 level rises. These changes are reversed with refeeding.[49] It is hoped that the enzymatic basis for these interesting transformations will emerge from future in vitro observations.

DISCORDANCE BETWEEN CIRCULATING T3 LEVEL AND CLINICAL STATE

As we have seen, it is clear evidence that T3 contributes a major proportion of the calorigenic potency of thyroid hormones. Nevertheless, many recent reports document a

Apparent Clinical Euthyroidism with Abnormal T3 Levels

Low T3 levels in the presence of the clinically euthyroid state have been reported in severe illness,[52] in the terminally ill,[51,52] in protein-caloric malnutrition,[53] anorexia nervosa,[54] in liver disease,[55,56] in kidney disease,[57] in the normal fetus,[58] in patients treated with large doses of steroids,[59] in fasting obese patients,[60] in patients with acute febrile illnesses,[61] and after operation.[62]

Hypothyroidism with Normal T3 Levels

On the other hand, Larsen[63] reported in 1972 that one-third of a group of hypothyroid patients with elevated TSH and low T4 levels had normal circulating levels of T3 and that for the most part those with normal T3 levels had mild disease. More recently he has made similar observations in milder cases of congenital hypothyroidism with borderline T4 levels that have been detected by routine screening procedures for congenital hypothyroidism. We have also observed normal T3 levels in some of our adult patients with mild hypothyroidism,[64] although the proportion of patients with normal T3 levels is far smaller in our experience (of the order of 5 percent or less).

One can explain the normal T3 level in terms of a preferential T3 production by the thyroid in response to a raised TSH or by hypothesizing a state of relative iodine deficiency in which damaged thyroid is unable to take up and utilize the requisite amount of iodide. (Iodine deficiency, as mentioned earlier, may cause increased T3 production in both man and experimental animals.) Another potential explanation for the increased T3:T4 ratio in incipient hypothyroidism might be increased peripheral conversion of T4 to T3, but this has been shown to be reduced in hypothyroid states.[65] The T3:T4 ratio is also increased after partial thyroidectomy or radioiodine treatment. Sterling et al.[65] reported 12 such patients who had low serum T4 levels even though they were clinically euthyroid. Nine of the patients had mildly raised TSH levels, and T3 levels were in the range of normal to low normal. Animal studies using subtotally thyroidectomized rats, in which more complete observations were possible, clearly showed that there was an increase in T3 production early in the development of hypothyroidism and that this increment could properly be ascribed to enhanced T3 secretion by the thyroid itself rather than to altered peripheral conversion.[67]

HYPERTHYROIDISM WITH NORMAL T3 LEVELS

Although a high T3 level has been reported to be the best single parameter for the diagnosis of hyperthyroidism, there have been reports of a number of purported cases of a new entity—so-called "T4 toxicosis." By definition, this syndrome of hyperthyroidism would occur if T4 level were raised in the presence of a normal T3. A number of possible cases have been reported.[68,69] All of these have been in elderly subjects, except for a single case reported by Turner et al.[70] in a 22-year-old otherwise healthy woman. She had clinical relapse of hyperthyroidism after a course of antithyroid drugs, and her T3 level was normal while her T4 was raised (unfortunately, no data on TBG levels were given).

Free thyroxine index (FTI) and T3 levels in 90 hyperthyroid patients were also reported by Hadden et al.[71] Seven patients had elevated T3 levels with normal FTI values, and 2 patients had normal T3 values with raised FTI values. Their conclusion was that both T3 toxicosis and T4 toxicosis exist.

A number of important points remain to be clarified before the existence of this syndrome can be unequivocally accepted. Britton[72] has found that contrary to previous observations[73] elevated T4 levels may be normal biochemical findings in elderly women. Moreover, physiologic decreases in T3 levels seen with aging and the effects of concomitant illness are well recognized. Finally, no studies of thyroidal secretion of T3 and T4 have been performed in these interesting patients; so we do not know the relative contributions of T3 and T4 to thyrometabolic states in the cases that have been described thus far.

CURRENT ROLE OF T3 IN DIAGNOSIS

The physiologic role of T3 (reviewed earlier in this chapter) seems securely established. In normal and hyperthyroid individuals T3 apparently contributes over two-thirds of the metabolic activity of thyroid hormones. Yet these are lingering questions. At present we cannot fully explain the many well-documented marked discordances that we have seen between metabolic status and circulating T3 levels. These questions must be carefully considered in defining the current role of T3 in the diagnosis of thyroid disease. The T3 level may be depressed in many euthyroid patients, e.g., those with concurrent illnesses[74,75] and the elderly.[21] Conversely, a normal T3 can be seen in mild hypothyroidism. Therefore T3 is of limited value in evaluating patients with hypothyroidism.

Raised T3 levels have been demonstrated in patients with hyperthyroidism, with little overlap with euthyroid patients,[15,21,76-77] and T3 toxicosis has been well documented.[23] Moreover, we have seen the usefulness of T3 determinations in evaluating patients with conventional hyperthyroidism prior to initiation of therapy, in predicting the likelihood of recurrence of the disease, and in gauging the success of therapy. T3 estimation is also helpful in thyrotoxic patients with low TBG levels.[79]

More recently, other workers have critically examined the diagnostic value of T3 in hyperthyroidism. Fifty-five patients suspected of having thyrotoxicosis were investigated by Marsden and McKerron.[37] Forty-six of the patients proved to be thyrotoxic, while 7 patients were euthyroid and 2 patients could not be classified. Analysis of their initial serum results showed that T3 level was superior to T4 level, to the resin uptake test, and to the FTI in predicting clinical outcome. Of 46 thyrotoxic patients, 8 patients (11 percent) had elevated T3 levels, with normal T4 level, FTI, and T3 resin uptake, fulfilling the criteria for T3 toxicosis. It is interesting that of these 8 patients, 3 had hot nodules, 3 were new cases of Graves' disease, and 2 were recurrent cases. Breaking the figures down further, the 3 patients with T3 toxicosis and hot nodules came from a total group of 6 patients, with the latter condition giving an incidence of 50 percent for T3 toxicosis in solitary hyperfunctioning nodules. Marsden found that borderline levels were much more common with T4 than with T3 in conventional hyperthyroidism. He stressed that T3 estimation was particularly valuable in certain clinical situations (i.e., the hyperfunctioning thyroid nodule and recurrent thyrotoxicosis) but he found it to be the best single thyroid function test in all hyperthyroid subjects studied. Other workers have also found T3 determinations valuable in hyperthyroidism.[80-82] Shalet et al.,[83] in a retrospective study, found that a significant number of patients considered thyrotoxic diagnosed only with the aid of serum T3 levels. In conclusion, on the basis of our own observations and those of others, we suggest that a T3 determination, which from all indications should become increasingly available over the next few years in this country and throughout the world, will prove to be a very useful diagnostic test and is warranted in all new patients suspected of having hyperthyroidism.

REFERENCES

1. Gross J, Pitt-Rivers R: The identification of 3:5:3'-L-triiodothyronine in man. Lancet 1:439, 1952
2. Roche J, Lissitzky S, Michel R: C R Acad Sci [D] (Paris) 1952
3. Maclagan NF, Bowden CH, Wilkinson JH: Detection of T4 and T3 in human plasma. Biochem J 67:5, 1957
4. Rupp JJ, Chavarria C, Paschkis KE, et al: The occurrence of T3 as the only circulating thyroid hormone. Ann Intern Med 51:359, 1959
5. Werner SC, Row VV, Radichevich I: Nontoxic nodular goiter with formation and release of a compound with the chromatographic mobility characteristic of T3. J Clin Endocrinol Metab 20:1373, 1960
6. Mack RE, Hart KT, Druet D, et al: An abnormality of thyroid hormone secretion. Am J Med 30:323, 1961
7. Rupp JJ, Paschkis KE: The changing pattern of evaluating iodinated amino acids in a case of thyrotoxicosis. Am J Med 30:472, 1961
8. Shimoaka K: Toxic adenoma of the thyroid with T3 as the principal circulating thyroid hormone. Acta Endocrinol (Kbh) 43:285, 1963
9. Czerniak P, Chaitchik S: Hypertriiodothyronism. Harefuah 66:218, 1964
10. Hollander CS: On the nature of circulating thyroid hormone: Clinical studies of T3 and T4 in serum using gas chromatographic methods. Trans Assoc Am Physicians 81:76, 1968
11. Hollander CS, Nihei N, Burday SZ: Abnormalities of T3 secretion in man: Clinical and pathophysiological studies using gas chromatographic techniques. Clin Res 27:236, 1969
12. Nauman JA, Nauman A, Werner SE: Total and free T3 in human serum. J Clin Invest 46:1346, 1967
13. Sterling K, Bellabarba D, Newman ES, et al: Determination of T3 concentration in human serum. J Clin Invest 48:1150, 1969
14. Brown DL, Ekins RP, Ellis SM, et al: Specific antibodies to triiodothyronine hormone. Nature 222:359, 1970
15. Mitsuma T, Nihei N, Gershengorn MC et al: Serum T3 measurements in human serum by radioimmunoassay with corroboration by gas liquid chromatography. J Clin Invest 50:2679, 1971
16. Lieblich J, Utiger RD: T3 radioimmunoassay. J Clin Invest 51:157, 1972
17. Larsen PR: Direct immunoassay of T3 in human serum. J Clin Invest 51:1939, 1972
18. Mitsuma T, Colucci J, Shenkman L, et al: Rapid radioimmunoassay for triiodothyronine and thyroxine in unextracted serum. Biochem Biophys Res Commun 46:2107, 1972
19. Chopra IJ, Solomon DH, Beall GN: Radioimmunoassay for measurement of T3 in human serum. J Clin Invest 50:2033, 1971
20. Surks MT, Schadlow AR, Oppenheimer JH: A new radioimmunoassay for plasma L-triiodothyronine: Measurements in thyroid disease and in patients maintained on hormonal replacement. J Clin Invest 51:3102, 1972
21. Rubenstein HA, Werner SC, Butler VP Jr: Progressive decrease in serum triiodothyronine concentrations with human aging: Radioimmunoassay following extraction of serum. J Clin Endocrinol Metab 37:247, 1973
22. Hollander CS, Shenkman L: Thyroxine and triiodothyronine, in Jaffe BM, Behrman HR (eds): Methods of Hormone Radioimmunoassay. New York Academic Press, 1974
23. Hollander CS, Mitsuma T, Nihei N, et al: Clinical and laboratory observations in cases of T3 toxicosis confirmed by radioimmunoassay. Lancet 1:609, 1972
24. Carter JN, Eastman CJ, Casey JH, et al: Triiodothyronine toxicosis. Med J Aust 8:229–233, 1975
25. Mitsuma T, Owens R, Shenkman L, et al: Hyperthyroidism due to isolated hypersecretion of triiodothyronine. J Pediatr 81:982, 1972
26. Sung LC, Cavaleri RR: T3 toxicosis due to metastatic thyroid carcinoma. J Clin Endocrinol Metab 36:215, 1973
27. Ahmed M, Doe RP, Nuhall FQ: Triiodothyronine Thyrotoxicosis following iodide ingestion — A case report. J Clin Endocrinol Metab 38:574–576, 1976
28. Ivy HK, Wahner HW, Gorman CA: T3 toxicosis. Arch Intern Med 128:529, 1971
29. Colantonio LA: T3 toxicosis-induction by dessiccated thryoid and imipramine. Am J Dis Child 128:396, 1976
30. Fairclough PD, Besser GM: Apathetic T3 toxicosis. Br Med J 1:364, 1974

31. Jacobs HS, Eastman CJ, Ekins RP, et al: Total and free T3 levels in thyroid storm and recurrent hyperthyroidism. Lancet 2:236, 1973
32. Tachibana T, Suzuki M: Proceedings: Case study of T3 toxicosis associated with periodic paralysis. Folia Endocrinol Jpn 50:396, 1976
33. Hollander CS, Mitsuma T, Kastin AJ, et al: Hypertriiodothyroninaemia as a premonitory manifestation of thyrotoxicosis. Lancet 2:731, 1971
34. Hollander CS, Shenkman L, Mitsuma T, et al: T3 toxicosis developing during antithyroid drug therapy for hyperthyroidism. Johns Hopkins Med J 131:184–188, 1972
35. Bellabarba D: Further observations on T3 toxicosis. Clin Res 20:421, 1972
36. Shenkman L, Mitsuma T, Blum M, et al: Recurrent hyperthyroidism presenting as T3 toxicosis. Ann Intern Med 20:421, 1972
37. Marsden P, McKerron CG: Serum T3 concentration in the diagnosis of hyperthyroidism. Clin Endocrinol 4:183, 1975
38. Hollander CS, Mitsuma T, Shenkman L, et al: T3 toxicosis in an iodine deficient area. Lancet 2:1276, 1972
39. Greer MA, Grimm Y, Studer H: Changes in thyroid secretion produced by inhibition of diiodotyrosine deiodinase. Endocrinology 83:405, 1968
40. Abrams GM, Larsen PR: T3 and T4 in the serum and thyroid gland of iodine deficient rats. J Clin Invest 52:2522, 1973
41. Taurog A, Porter J, Thio D, et al: Nature of the I^{131} compounds released into the thyroid veins of rabbits, dogs, cats before and after TSH administration. Endocrinology 74:902, 1964
42. Gross J: T3 in relation to thyroid physiology. Recent Prog Horm Res 10:109, 1954
43. Pitt-Rivers R, Stanbury JB, Rapp B: Conversion of T4 to T3 in vivo. J Clin Endocrinol Metab 15:616, 1955
44. Lassiter WE, Stanbury JB: The in vivo conversion of T4 to T3. J Clin Endocrinol Metab 18:903, 1958
45. Chopra IJ: An assessment of daily production and significance of thyroidal secretion of reverse T3 in man. J Clin Invest 8:32, 1976
46. Griffiths RS, Black EG, Hoffenberg R: Measurement of serum 3, 3', 5'-T3 (reverse T3) with comments on its derivation. Clin Endocrinol 5:679–685, 1976
47. Herrmann J, Lehr HL, Kroll HT, et al: Excessive peripheral conversion of thyroxine (T4) to triiodothyronine in the pathogenesis of hyperthyroidism. Dtsch Med Wochenschr 100:2319, 1975
48. Wenzel KW, Meinhold H: T3/rT3 balance in thyroxine metabolism. Lancet 2:413, 1975
49. Vagenakis AG, Burger A, Portnay G, et al: Diversion of peripheral thyroxine metabolism from activating to inactivating pathways during complete fasting. J Clin Endocrinol Metab 41:191, 1975
50. Carter, JN, Eastman CJ, Corcoran JM, et al: Effect of severe, chronic illness on thyroid function. Lancet 2:971, 1971
51. Reichlin S, Bottinger J, Negad I, et al: Tissue thyroid hormone concentration of rat and man determined by radioimmunoassay: Biological significance. Mt. Sinai J Med NY 40:502, 1973
52. Sullivan PRC, Bollinger JA, Reichlin S: Selective deficiency of tissue triiodothyronine. J Clin Invest 52:83a, 1973
53. Chopra IJ, Smith SR: Circulating thyroid hormone and thyrotropin in adult patients with protein-calorie malnutrition. J Clin Endocrinol Metab 40:221, 1975
54. Moshang T Jr, Parks JS, Baker L, et al: Low serum triiodothyronine in patients with anorexia nervosa. J Clin Endocrinol Metab 40:470, 1975
55. Chopra IJ, Solomon DH, Chopra U, et al: Alteration in circulating thyroid hormones and thyrotropin in hepatic cirrhosis. J Clin Endocrinol Metab 39:501, 1974
56. Nomura S, Chambers MW Jr, Buck M, et al: Conversion of T4 to T3 in liver patients. Clin Res 22:62, 1974
57. Chopra IJ, Chopra U, Smith SR: Reciprocal changes in serum concentration of 3-3'-5' triiodothyronine (reverse T3) and 3-3'-5 triiodothyronine (T3) in systemic illness.
58. Fisher DA, Dussault JH, Hebel CT, et al: Serum and thyroid gland triiodothyronine in the human fetus. J Clin Endocrinol Metab 36:397, 1973
59. Duick DS, Warren DW, Nicoloff ST, et al: Effect of single dose dexamethasone on the concentration of serum triiodothyronine in man. J Clin Endocrinol Metab 39:1151, 1974
60. Spaulding SW, Chopra IJ, Sherwin RS, et al: Effect of caloric restriction and dietary composition on serum T3 and reverse T3 in man. J Clin Endocrinol Metab 42:197, 1976
61. Chopra IJ, Chopra U, Smith SR, et al: Reciprocal changes in serum concentration of reverse T3 and LT3 in systemic illnesses. J Clin Endocrinol Metab 41:1043, 1973
62. Burr WA, Griffiths RS, Black EG, et al: Serum triiodothyronine and reverse triiodothyronine concentrations after surgical operations. Lancet 2:1272, 1975
63. Larsen PR: T3. Review of recent studies of its physiology and pathophysiology in man. Metabolism 21:1073, 1972
64. Mitsuma T, Nihei N, Gershengorn M, et al: Serum triiodothyronine measurements in human serum by radioimmunoassay with corroboration

by gas-liquid chromatography. J Clin Invest 50:2679, 1971
65. Inada M, Kasagi K, Kurata S, et al: Estimation of thyroxine and triiodothyronine distribution and of the conversion rate of thyroxine to triiodothyronine in man. J Clin Invest 55:1337, 1975
66. Sterling KM, Brenner ES, Newman WD, et al: The significance of T3 in maintenance of euthyroid status after treatment of hyperthyroidism. J Clin Endocrinol Metab 33:729, 1971
67. Imai Y, Kataoka K, Hollander CS: Sequential alteration in serum triiodothyronine, thyroxine and thyrotropin levels in developing hypothyroidism, in: Proceedings of 7th International Thyroid Conference. Excerpta Med Int Congr Ser 378:523, 1975
68. Kirkegaard C, Sirosback-Nielson K, Triis TH, et al: Does T4 toxicosis exist? Lancet 1:868, 1975
69. Turner JG, Brownlie BE, Sadler WA: Does T4 toxicosis exist? Lancet 1:407, 1975
70. Turner JG, Brownlie BE, Sadler WA, et al: Does T4 toxicosis exist? Lancet 1:1292, 1975
71. Hadden DR, McMaster A, Bell TK, et al: Does T4 toxicosis exist? Lancet 1:754, 1975
72. Britton KE, Quinn V, Ellis SM: Is T4 toxicosis a normal documented finding in elderly women? Lancet 2:141, 1975
73. Gregerman RI, Bierman EL: Mechanism of altered metabolic rate of T4 and T3 in Williams RH (ed): Textbook of Endocrinology. Philadelphia, WB Saunders, 1974
74. Bermudez F, Surks MI, Oppenheimer JH: High incidence of decreased serum triiodothyronine concentration in patients with nonthyroidal disease. J Clin Endocrinol Metab 41:2240, 1975
75. Carter JN, Eastman CJ, Corcoran JM, et al: Effect of severe, chronic illness on thyroid function. Lancet 2:971, 1971
76. Larsen PR: T3—Review of recent studies of its physiology and pathophysiology in man. Metabolism 21:1073, 1972
77. Lieblich J, Utiger RD: T3 radioimmunoassay. J Clin Invest 51:157, 1972
78. Chopra, IJ, Solomon DH, Beall GN: Radioimmunoassay for measurement of T3 in human serum. J Clin Invest 50:2033, 1971
79. Wahner HW, Emstander RF, Gorman CA: Thyroid overactivity and TBG deficiency simulating T3 toxicosis. J Clin Endocrinol Metab 33 93, 1971
80. Hesch RD, Emrich D, von zur Muhlen A: Value of radioimmunoassay of triiodothyronine and thyrotropic hormone in diagnosis of thyroid disease. Dtsch Med Wochenschr 100:805, 1975
81. Nouel JP, Brunelle P, Segond G: Le dosage de la triiodothyronine serique en pathologie thyrodienne bilan de deux années d'experience. Ann Endocrinol (Paris) 35:269, 1974
82. Peyrin JO, Bomet H, Roux D: Premiers resultats comparés aux autres paramètres seriques du dosage radioimmunologique de T3 en pathologie. Ann Endocrinol (Paris) 35:271, 1974
83. Shalet SM, Beardwell CG, Lamb AM, et al: Value of routine serum T3 estimation in the diagnosis of thyrotoxicosis. Lancet 1:1008, 1975

Robert G. Dluhy

4
Diagnosis and Treatment of Adrenocortical Insufficiency

The adrenal cortex synthesizes three classes of steroid hormones: glucocorticoids, mineralocorticoids, and androgens. These hormones are secreted by different zones of the adrenal cortex, while the control of secretion is regulated by different tropic factors. Glucocorticoids (cortisol) are secreted by the zona fasciculata, while androgens (predominantly dehydroepiandrosterone) are produced in the zona reticularis. The control of glucocorticoid and adrenocortical androgen secretion is predominantly regulated by pituitary adrenocorticotropic hormone (ACTH). On the other hand, the mineralocorticoid aldosterone is secreted by the zona glomerulosa. Aldosterone secretion is regulated by multiple factors, predominantly the renin-angiotensin system and potassium.[1]

It logically follows that adrenocortical insufficiency may result from primary disease or dysfunction of the adrenal cortex, or insufficiency may be secondary to deficiencies of regulating tropic factors, such as ACTH or renin and angiotensin. Accordingly, adrenocortical insufficiency syndromes may reflect diseases involving all zones of the cortex, or the hormonal deficiency may be selective. For example, Addison's disease is a primary adrenal insufficiency syndrome involving all three zones of the cortex, while selective primary adrenal deficiency states include the congenital adrenal hyperplasia syndromes as well as the syndrome of isolated hypoaldosteronism. On the other hand, adrenal insufficiency secondary to hypothalamic-pituitary ACTH deficiency results in subnormal cortisol and adrenal androgen output, while aldosterone secretion is usually preserved by the renin-angiotensin system.

The etiologies of adrenocortical insufficiency states are varied, ranging from pituitary tumors to adrenal gland atrophy and destruction. Documentation of secondary adrenocortical insufficiency should logically lead to a careful evaluation of all pituitary tropic hormones. More than 90 percent of the adrenal glands must be destroyed before clinical signs of insufficiency appear. In 90 percent of these cases primary adrenal insufficiency is caused by bilateral tuberculosis or, more commonly, by bilateral idiopathic atrophy. Patients with idiopathic or autoimmune adrenal atrophy often have circulating levels of adrenal antibodies, as well as antibodies to thyroid, parathyroid, and gastric mucosal tissue.[2] Accordingly, it has been found that patients with idiopathic primary adrenal insufficiency have a higher incidence of Hashimoto's thyroiditis and thyroid failure (Schmidt's syndrome).[3] Pernicious anemia also occurs more frequently in patients with Addison's disease, while hypoparathyroidism and adrenal atrophy also occur together, sometimes in association with systemic moniliasis.[4] Of recent interest are reports documenting that so-called autoimmune endocrine deficiency states occur significantly more frequently in patients with certain leukocyte antigens.

In 1855 Thomas Addison published his classic description of chronic adrenocortical insufficiency: "The leading and characteristic features of the morbid state to which I would direct attention are anemia, general languor and debility, remarkable feebleness of the heart's action, irritability of the stomach, and a peculiar change of colour in the skin, occurring in connection with a diseased condition of the suprarenal capsules."[5] Thus this disease should be suspected from a triad of symptoms: unexplained weakness and fatigue, hypotension, and melanosis (Table 4–1). Glucocorticoid insufficiency results in weakness, nonspecific gastrointestinal illness (anorexia, nausea, vomiting, abdominal pain), and impaired tolerance to stress. Lack of cortisol also results in high blood concentrations of ACTH and melanocyte-stimulating hormone (MSH); MSH elevations result in mucocutaneous hyperpigmentation, particularly of exposed points such as elbows and creases of the hand. Normally pigmented areas (such as the areolae) darken, and melanotic patches appear on the mucous membranes, while some patients develop dark freckles and irregular areas of vitiligo. Diminished mineralocorticoid activity leads to dehydration, weight loss, and the characteristic chemistry triad of azotemia, hyponatremia and hyperkalemia. In female patients decreased adrenal androgen production may be associated with loss of axillary and pubic hair.

The symptoms of adrenal insufficiency as a consequence of ACTH deficiency may be indistinguishable from those of Addison's disease, but ACTH and MSH levels are low rather than high. Therefore mucocutaneous hyperpigmentation is absent, but it is emphasized that melanosis is not a universal finding in patients with Addison's disease. Since aldosterone secretion is preserved in patients with ACTH deficiency, severe dehydration and the characteristic blood electrolyte pattern of hyponatremia-hyperkalemia are not observed. Patients with secondary adrenocortical insufficiency also frequently have symptoms and signs of multiple pituitary tropic hormone deficiencies. On the other hand, steroid-induced adrenal insufficiency is associated with selective ACTH deficiency.

Adrenal crisis is a rapid and overwhelming intensification of chronic adrenal insufficiency. High fever, severe hypotension or vascular collapse, and nausea and vomiting characterize this syndrome. Severe electrolyte abnormalities may be present if mineralocorticoid secretion is also impaired. It is emphasized, however, that adrenal crisis is seen secondary to cortisol insufficiency alone. Crisis is usually precipitated in patients with adrenal insufficiency by severe stress, most commonly intercurrent infection, trauma, or surgery.

The diagnosis of adrenal insufficiency is established by a subnormal functional response of the adrenal cortex following ACTH stimulation. Basal urine or blood levels of cortisol and cortisol metabolites are not diagnostic because of the overlap between low and normal levels. Following the documentation of inadequate adrenal reserve, appropriate tests should be employed to distinguish primary from secondary adrenocortical insufficiency.

A common outpatient test for adrenal insufficiency is the measurement of the plasma cortisol response following administration of 0.25 mg (25 units) of α^{1-24}-corticotropin (cosyntropin) intramuscularly,[6,7] The normal response is a doubling of basal cortisol levels within 30 to 60 min. Additional criteria indicate that the 30- or 60-min cortisol

Table 4-1
Symptoms of Adrenal Cortical Hypofunction

1. Unexplained weakness
2. Hypotension
3. Increased pigmentation
4. Unexplained weight loss
5. Hypoglycemic manifestations
6. Unexplained gastrointestinal symptoms
7. Poor response to stress

value should show an increment above basal levels of 7 µg/dl or 11 µg/dl, respectively, or that the 30-min level should exceed 18 µg/dl. Although aldosterone secretion in normal man is primarily regulated by potassium and the renin-angiotensin system, ACTH is also a potent acute stimulus.[1] In normal subjects on uncontrolled dietary sodium intake the mean increment of plasma aldosterone level above control at 30 min following intramuscular administration of 0.25 mg of cosyntropin was 14 ng/dl (range 4–29 ng/dl)[8] (Table 4–2). It is likely that differences in diet explain the range of responses in normal subjects, since it is known that dietary sodium intake markedly alters aldosterone responsiveness to ACTH stimulation.[9]

Standard intravenous ACTH testing is accomplished by a continuous 8-hr infusion (8 A.M. to 4 P.M.) of 0.25 mg synthetic ACTH (cosyntropin) for 2 or 3 consecutive days.[10] Alternatively, lyophilized pituitary ACTH (40 units) may be used, but synthetic ACTH is recommended because of its greater purity. Daily urine collections are tested for creatinine and 17-hydroxycorticoid and 17-ketosteroid levels. In normal subjects the average increment in urine 17-hydroxycorticoids on the first day of testing is 15 mg/24 hr (25 mg/24 hr on the second infusion day). Alternatively, blood cortisol levels may be measured at the beginning and end of the 8-hr infusion. Normal subjects exhibit an increment above control of 10–20 µg/dl during the first hour, while the blood cortisol increment should exceed 20 µg/dl by the eighth hour (range 20–40 µg/dl).

Table 4-2
Plasma Aldosterone Response after Administration of Cosyntropin in Normal Persons and Patients with Adrenal Hypofunction

	No. of Subjects	Base line (ng/100 ml)	30 Minutes after Cosyntropin† (ng/100 ml)	Increment (ng/100 ml)
Normal persons	12	14* (1–40)	28* (5–55)	14* (4–29)
Primary adrenal insufficiency	5	2 (0–4)	2 (0–4)	0 (0–1)
Secondary adrenal insufficiency				
Steroid-treated	6	18 (3–25)	44 (20–62)	26 (3–43)
Pituitary-insufficient	6	5 (0–8)	11 (5–16)	7 (5–10)

*Mean values; range in parentheses
†Intramuscular injection, 0.25 mg (25 units).

Pituitary ACTH reserve is commonly assessed with the use of the drug metyrapone, an agent that selectively inhibits the enzyme 11β-hydroxylase in the adrenal gland.[11] As a result, 11-deoxycortisol levels accumulate, while blood levels of cortisol decline. The anterior pituitary responds to declining cortisol levels by releasing increased quantities of ACTH in an attempt to return cortisol levels toward normal. As a result of the enzymatic blockade, increasing quantities of metabolites of 11-deoxycortisol appear in the urine, where they are measured as 17-hydroxycorticoids. Metyrapone is administered orally every 4 hr in doses of 750 mg over 24–48 hr; urinary collections are obtained daily for 17-hydroxycorticosteroids. The normal response is at least doubling of basal 17-hydroxycorticoid excretion. An alternative test of pituitary ACTH reserve may be accomplished by insulin tolerance testing.[12] From 0.05 to 0.1 unit of crystalline insulin per kilogram of body weight is given as a bolus intravenously in order to reduce blood sugar levels at least 50% below control. In response to the stimulus of hypoglycemia, blood ACTH and subsequently cortisol levels rise promptly. The normal response is a doubling of cortisol levels above control at the time of peak blood sugar reduction, usually within 30–60 min following insulin administration. It is stressed that abnormal metyrapone or insulin tolerance testing does not establish a diagnosis of pituitary ACTH deficiency, since it must be demonstrated that the adrenal glands are capable of being stimulated by ACTH.

An abnormal response to standard ACTH testing does not distinguish between primary and secondary adrenocortical insufficiency. In general, primary adrenal insufficiency is associated with very low levels of cortisol (less than 5μg/dl) that fail to rise following ACTH stimulation. On the other hand, secondary adrenocortical insufficiency is associated with adrenal atrophy, but an increment in adrenal glucocorticoid secretion can be elicited following prolonged ACTH stimulation. Thus patients with pituitary insufficiency or subjects receiving long-term steroid therapy exhibit a staircase response, with successive increments in steroid secretion if standard 8-hr ACTH testing is continued for 4–5 days. Alternatively, a continuous intravenous ACTH infusion over 24–48 hr can accurately distinguish between normal adrenocortical function, primary adrenal insufficiency, and secondary adrenocortical failure, thus shortening the period of ACTH testing.[13] Synthetic ACTH (cosyntropin), 0.25 mg/12 hr, is infused continuously over 48 hr. Normal subjects will excrete urinary 17-hydroxycorticoids at a rate greater than 27 mg/24 hr on the first infusion day and greater than 47 mg/24 hr on the second infusion day. Subjects with primary adrenocortical insufficiency show little response, excreting less than 3 mg/24 hr on the first infusion day and less than 4 mg/24 hr on the second infusion day. Patients with secondary adrenocortical insufficiency excrete more than 4 mg/24 hr on the first infusion day and 10 mg/24 hr on the second infusion day.

Aldosterone secretion following ACTH stimulation should also be useful in differential diagnosis, since the production of aldosterone is maintained in patients with secondary but not primary adrenal insufficiency. Primary adrenal insufficiency is associated with fixed low rates of aldosterone secretion, and mineralocorticoid replacement therapy is ordinarily necessary. Although aldosterone secretion is preserved in patients with secondary adrenocortical insufficiency, diminished responsiveness following acute stimulation is the rule.[14] Following intramuscular administration of 0.25 mg of cosyntropin, normal individuals exhibit increments of plasma aldosterone, on the average, 14 ng/dl (range 4–20 ng/dl) above control at 30 min[8] (Table 4–2). In contrast, patients with primary adrenal failure exhibit plasma aldosterone levels under 4 ng/dl that fail to rise following ACTH stimulation (Fig. 4–1). In patients with pituitary insufficiency the mean plasma aldosterone increment above control following intramuscular cosyntropin injection is 7 ng/dl (range 5–10 ng/dl). Thus a control plasma aldosterone level under 5 ng/dl that fails

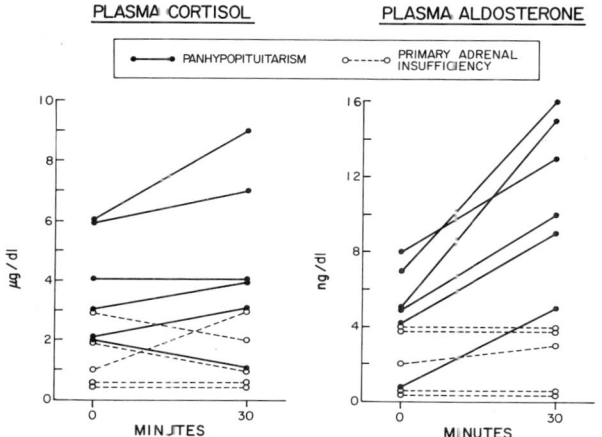

Fig. 4-1. Plasma cortisol and aldosterone responses after intramuscular administration of 0.25 mg (25 units) cosyntropin in patients with primary adrenal insufficiency (5) and patients with panhypopituitarism (6).

to rise following ACTH stimulation strongly supports a diagnosis of primary adrenocortical insufficiency. In contrast with the aldosterone responses in normal subjects, the lower stimulated-aldosterone values in patients with pituitary insufficiency indirectly support a role for pituitary factors in the normal maintenance of aldosterone secretion.

Patients with primary adrenocortical insufficiency (Addison's disease) ordinarily require replacement glucocorticoid and mineralocorticoid therapy.[15,16] Cortisone (or hydrocortisone) is the mainstay of treatment; ordinarily the cortisone dosage varies from 12.5 to 37.5 mg daily, while hydrocortisone (30 mg daily) and prednisone (7.5 mg daily) may also be used for substitution therapy. The larger proportion of the dose is usually taken in the early morning, with the remainder in the early or late afternoon. Since cortisol is secreted in normal subjects in relation to body surface area, it stands to reason that large individuals will require greater replacement doses as compared to lean or small subjects. As a rule, 10–12 mg of cortisol are secreted in normal subjects per square meter per day.

Mineralocorticoid replacement therapy is usually accomplished by daily oral administration of the potent salt-retaining hormone 9α-fluorohydrocortisone.[15,16] The daily dose usually ranges between 0.1 mg and 0.2 mg, but the requirement is inversely related to the average dietary intake of sodium. Small doses of androgen may also be used to advantage in female patients if libido and general sense of well-being remain below normal after glucocorticoid and mineralocorticoid therapies have been instituted. A starting dose would be 25–50 mg of testosterone enanthate in oil intramuscularly each month, but patients should be surveyed closely to avoid masculinizing side effects.

All patients with adrenocortical insufficiency should be carefully educated in regard to their disease and should carry medical identification. They should also be instructed in the parenteral self-administration of steroids, and they should automatically increase their dosage of cortisone or hydrocortisone during intercurrent illness. For mild febrile illness, patients should ordinarily double their replacement glucocorticoid intake. Extra sodium should be added to the diet, or the dose of mineralocorticoid replacement should be increased, during periods of excessive exercise with sweating, during hot weather, or during periods of gastrointestinal upset.

Adrenal crisis patients or addisonian patients undergoing major stress, such as general anesthesia, demand maximal glucocorticoid therapeutic schedules. Treatment is directed toward rapid elevation of circulating glucocorticoid levels to approximate the maximal adrenal output of normal subjects (10 mg of cortisol per hour). Hence an intravenous infusion of 1000 ml of 5 percent glucose in normal saline containing 100 mg of hydrocortisone is administered at a rate of 100 ml/hr. If the condition is extreme, such as adrenal crisis, 100 mg of hydrocortisone are given rapidly within the first few minutes intravenously, followed by a continuous infusion of glucocorticoid as outlined above. In addition, sodium and water deficits should be replaced as indicated by the estimated state of hydration. With large doses of hydrocortisone, mineralocorticoid replacement therapy is not indicated; however, when cortisol dosage is reduced below 100 mg/24 hr, supplementary salt-retaining hormone therapy is usually necessary. On the day of major surgical stress or adrenal crisis, the total cortisol dose should be 250–300 mg/24 hr as a continuous infusion. On subsequent days, depending on the patient's condition, steroid dosage may be tapered in 20 percent decrements daily. A fraction of the total steroid dose may be given intramuscularly as cortisone acetate to ensure continued glucocorticoid therapy if the intravenous infusion should be interrupted.

Isolated aldosterone deficiency has been reported as a result of a congenital biosynthetic defect or, more commonly, in association with hyporeninism.[17] All patients with hypoaldosteronism fail to increase aldosterone output following salt restriction. Hyponatremia and hyperkalemia are common to all hypoaldosterone syndromes; renin levels are elevated in congenital or acquired biosynthetic defects, while levels are reduced in the syndrome of hyporeninism. Reversal of the signs of salt-wasting may be achieved by administration of potent mineralocorticoids (0.1–0.3 mg 9α-fluorohydrocortisone daily). The rapid ACTH test with plasma aldosterone levels is useful in the diagnosis of hypoaldosteronism.[8] In congenital biosynthetic defects, as well as hypoaldosteronism associated with hyporeninism, plasma aldosterone levels fail to rise normally following ACTH stimulation.

REFERENCES

1. Williams GH, Dluhy RG: Aldosterone biosynthesis: Interrelationship of regulatory factors. Am J Med 53:595, 1972
2. Blizzard R, Kyle M: Studies of the adrenal antigens and antibodies in Addison's disease. J Clin Invest 42:1653, 1963
3. Carpenter CCJ, Solomon N, Silverberg SC, et al: Schmidt's syndrome (thyroid and adrenal insufficiency): A review of the literature and a report of fifteen new cases including ten instances of coexistent diabetes mellitus. Medicine 43:153, 1964
4. Whitaker J, Landing BH, Esselborn VM, et al: The syndrome of familial juvenile hypoadrenocorticalism, hypoparathyroidism, and superficial moniliasis. J Clin Endocrinol Metab 16:1374, 1956
5. Addison T: The Constitutional and Local Effects of Disease of the Suprarenal Capsules. London, D Highley, 1855
6. Wood JB, Frankland AW, James VHT, et al: A rapid test of adrenocortical function. Lancet 1:243, 1965
7. Greig WR, Browning MCK, Boyle JA, et al: Effect of the synthetic polypeptide beta 1–24 (Synacthen) on adrenocortical function. J Clin Endocrinol Metab 34:411, 1966
8. Dluhy RG, Himathongkam T, Greenfield M: Rapid ACTH test with plasma aldosterone levels: Improved diagnostic discrimination. Ann Intern Med 80:693, 1974
9. Tucci JR, Espiner EA, Jagger PI, et al: ACTH stimulation of aldosterone secretion in normal subjects and in patients with chronic adrenocortical insufficiency. J Clin Endocrinol Metab 27:568, 1967
10. Jenkins D, Forsham PH, Laidlaw JE, et al: Use of ACTH in the diagnosis of adrenal cortical insufficiency. Am J Med 18:3, 1955
11. Liddle GW, Estep HL, Kendall JW, et al: Clini-

cal application of a new test of pituitary reserve. J Clin Endocrinol Metab 19:875, 1959
12. Landon J, Wynn V, James VHT: The adrenocortical response in insulin-induced hypoglycemia. J Endocrinol 27:183, 1963
13. Rose LI, Williams GH, Jagger PI, et al: The 48-hour adrenocorticotropin test for adrenocortical insufficiency. Ann Intern Med 73:49, 1970
14. Williams GH, Rose LI, Dluhy RG, et al: Aldosterone response to sodium restriction and ACTH stimulation in panhypopituitarism. J Clin Endocrinol Metab 32:27, 1971
15. Dluhy RG, Newmark SR, Lauler DP, et al: Pharmacology and chemistry of adrenal glucocorticoids, in DL Azarnoff (ed): Steroid Therapy. Philadelphia, WB Saunders, 1975, p 1
16. Williams GH, Dluhy RG, Thorn GW: Diseases of the adrenal cortex, in Thorn GW, Adams RD, Braunwald E (eds): Harrison's Principles of Internal Medicine (ed 8). New York, McGraw-Hill, 1977, p 520
17. Biglieri EG: Isolated hypoaldosteronism in adults: A renin deficiency syndrome. N Engl J Med 287:573, 1972

David H.P. Streeten,
Theodore G. Dalakos, and
Gunnar H. Anderson, Jr.

5
Diagnosis and Treatment of Cushing's Syndrome

Cushing's syndrome results from excessive cortisol action on tissues, with or without features of androgen excess. Any one or several of the classic symptoms (obesity, fatigue, headaches, backaches, psychic symptoms) may be absent The most reliable signs are obesity in the face, neck, and shoulder girdle areas, hirsutism, cutaneous erythema and ecchymoses, and hypertension. Steroid measurements are essential for diagnosis in most instances. The best screening procedures are measurements of urinary 17-hydroxy-corticosteroid (17-OHCS) excretion per gram of creatinine (normal 2–6.5 mg/g creatinine) and measurements of urinary free cortisol (normal 10–90 µg/day) and plasma cortisol at 8 A.M. after 1 mg of dexamethasone at 11 P.M. (normal <5 µg/dl). For definitive diagnosis of this important disorder, at least three of the following criteria should be met: (1) urinary 17-OHCS (mean of two or three determinations) > 6.5 mg/g creatinine; (2) urinary free cortisol > 90 µg/day; (3) plasma cortisol (mean of 4 to 48 measurements at all times of the day and night) > 20 µg/dl, (4) cortisol secretion rate > 19 mg/g urinary creatinine; (5) on second day of dexamethasone (5 µg/kg/6 hr), urinary 17-OHCS > 1 mg/g creatinine. Failure of urinary 17-OHCS to fall by more than 50 percent on the second day of a larger dose of dexamethasone (2 mg every 6 hr) almost invariably indicates adrenal, pituitary (rarely), or ectopic ACTH-producing tumor. Plasma ACTH measurements may be helpful in differentiating these disorders. Simultaneous adrenal vein (bilateral) and peripheral vein plasma cortisol concentrations are often useful in this differentiation and in determining the side of an adrenal adenoma or carcinoma. Metyrapone and ACTH administrations are of more limited value.

Treatment of an adrenal adenoma is surgical. Adrenal carcinoma should be excised and usually treated with irradiation or O, P'-DDD therapy. Ectopic ACTH-producing neoplasms (usually malignant) should be looked for and excised, if this is practicable. Pituitary adenomas (when recognizable by enlargement of the sella) should usually be excised. Patients with bilateral adrenal hyperplasia may be treated in various ways, with

---

Supported by a Graduate Training Grant in Endocrinology (AM 07146) from the National Institute of Arthritis, Metabolism and Digestive Diseases and by a Clinical Research Center Grant (RR 00229) from the Division of Research Facilities and Resources, USPHS.

individualization of the therapeutic choice from among pituitary irradiation (in mild cases, especially in women desiring future pregnancies), pituitary ablation (excision, cryosurgery, ^{90}Y implants, heavy-particle irradiation), bilateral adrenalectomy (especially in very severe cases) with or without pituitary irradiation, and O,P'-DDD therapy. Educating the patient and her spouse to the need for increased steroid dosage if and when stresses occur after surgical therapy of Cushing's syndrome is of great importance.

Cushing's syndrome is the disorder that results from persistently excessive action of cortisol (i.e., hypercortisolism) over a period of months or years, with or without a concomitant excess of other adrenal steroid activity. Patients with severe forms of the syndrome are easily recognizable because of the presence of the symptoms and signs originally described by Cushing[1] in 1932: headaches, backaches, weakness, amenorrhea (in females), impotence (in males), hirsutism, obesity (face, neck, and abdomen, but sparing the limbs), purple striae of the abdominal wall and thighs, hypertension, hyperglycemia, and osteoporosis. In such instances all of the usual laboratory tests provide strongly confirmatory evidence, so that diagnosis is straightforward. As in most endocrinopathies, however, Cushing's syndrome is far more frequently seen in milder forms, with several of the features seen in the more severely afflicted individuals being lacking. Occasionally[2] patients may present no symptoms at all, and in a recent series[2] of 17 patients the incidences of the most common features were as shown in Table 5–1.

It has been pointed out[3,4] that in children with hypercortisolism the classic symptoms of Cushing's syndrome may be largely absent, with stunting of growth being the only complaint. In these and other circumstances where clinical features are inconclusive, laboratory findings become all-important. Of the laboratory procedures available, some are simple enough to be used as outpatient screening tests: e.g., measurement of urinary excretion of 17-hydroxycorticosteroids (17-OHCS) per gram of urinary creatinine and measurements of urinary free cortisol excretion and plasma cortisol at 8 A.M. after administration of 1 mg of dexamethasone at 11 P.M. the night before.[5,6] Other tests usually require hospitalization for their performance, and they are considered more nearly definitive indicators of the presence or absence of hypercortisolism: plasma cortisol concentrations measured repeatedly at all times of the day and night, 2-day dexamethasone suppression studies, and measurement of cortisol secretion rate. The reliability of these diagnostic tests may be illustrated by the results obtained in studies on 34 patients in Syracuse, New York over the past 16 years, all with conclusive evidence for the presence of pathologic hypercortisolism. All of these studies were performed at the Clinical Research Center of the Upstate Medical Center.

LABORATORY PROCEDURES

Urinary 17-OHCS per Gram of Creatinine

The advantages of expressing urinary 17-OHCS excretion as a function of creatinine excretion were first described in 1969.[2] Experience since then has fully substantiated the reliability of the results as indicators of the presence of normal or abnormal amounts of cortisol metabolites in the urine, as long as the measurements are made on at least two or three 24-hr urines (vide infra).

Table 5–1
Incidences of Common Symptoms and Signs of Cushing's Syndrome

Symptom	Incidence
Facial rounding	100%
Trunkal obesity	88%
Hirsutism in women	84%
Diabetic glucose tolerance	80%
Fatigue	71%
Weakness	65%
Excessive ease of bruising	65%
Osteoporosis	65%
Menstruation irregular or absent in premenopausal women	63%
Hypertension	59%
Headaches	59%
Backaches	53%
Purple striae	53%
Ankle edema	53%

Plasma Cortisol Concentration.

Krieger et al.[7] and Hellman et al.[8] have shown that in normal subjects plasma cortisol concentration fluctuates widely throughout the day and night, apparently because of episodic secretion of ACTH by the pituitary. Similar episodic changes in plasma cortisol concentration have been shown to occur in patients with Cushing's syndrome.[9,10] Measurements of plasma cortisol concentration every half hour for 24 hr in 2 patients with Cushing's syndrome and in a normal subject are shown in Figure 5–1. It is evident that plasma cortisol concentrations in the patient with severe hypercortisolism (uppermost curve) were consistently well above the normal values in all 48 determinations. The patient with mild hypercortisolism showed episodic variations in plasma cortisol concentration, as did the normal subject, with many determinations overlapping or being slightly lower than those in the normal subject. Moreover, in single determinations of plasma cortisol in patients who were subsequently shown not to have hypercortisolism, we have frequently found values well over 30 or even over 40 μg/dl that fell to clearly normal levels when the stress of an initial office visit or hospital admission had subsided. Thus it is clear that no reliance can be placed on the diagnostic significance of any one or two measurements of plasma cortisol concentration in patients suspected of having hypercortisolism. However, there seems to be a tendency for plasma cortisol concentration to be higher in the patient with mild hypercortisolism than in the normal subject. For this reason a comparison was made between the means of between 4 and 48 determinations evenly spaced throughout the 24 hr (e.g., every 6 hr or every half hour) in 25 patients with strong collateral evidence of Cushing's syndrome, 15 subjects with normal adrenal function, and 10 patients with primary or secondary adrenal insufficiency (Fig. 5–2). It is evident that mean plasma cortisol concentration throughout the day and night was above 20 μg/dl in all 25 patients with hypercortisolism and was between 4.5 and 15.8 μg/dl in all subjects with normal adrenal function, except for 1 individual (25.4 μg/dl). This patient (A, Fig. 5–2) was anxious and worried and was clearly much disturbed by the half-hour collections of

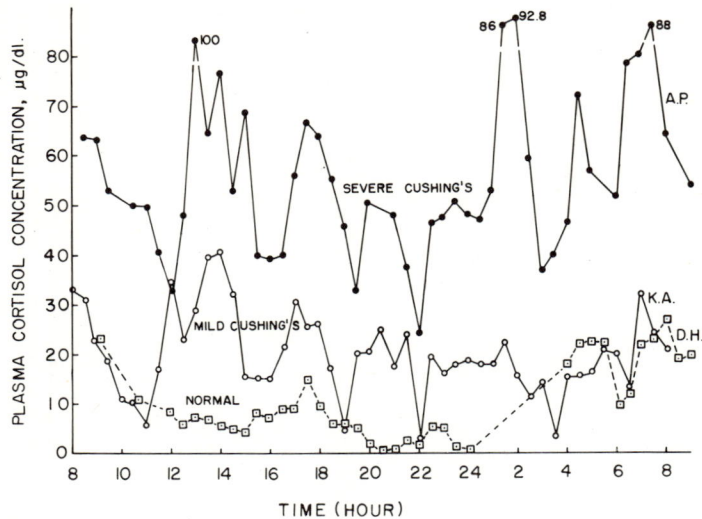

Fig. 5-1. Half-hourly measurements of plasma cortisol concentrations in 2 patients with hypercortisolism and 1 normal subject showing the overlapping of individual results obtained in the patient with mild hypercortisolism and the normal individual.

blood, in spite of the fact that these were made (as in all the depicted studies) without pain, by aspiration through an indwelling venous cannula, the patency of which was maintained by filling it with dilute (1:1000) heparin solution between samplings. With the exception of the measurements in this 1 patient, therefore, mean plasma cortisol concentration always separated patients with hypercortisolism from patients with normal adrenal function. Adrenal insufficiency was associated with mean plasma cortisol concentrations almost invariably below 4.4 μ/dl, the lowest normal level by the competitive protein binding method used in these studies.

Dexamethasone Suppression Tests

OVERNIGHT DEXAMETHASONE SUPPRESSION

The simple screening procedure introduced by Nugent et al.,[5] and Pavlatos et al.,[6] in which plasma cortisol concentration is measured at 8 A.M. after taking 1 mg of dexamethasone at 11 P.M. the previous night, has become very popular and widely used, in spite of the fact that its reliability has never been established. Although this procedure has been shown to give abnormal results in many patients with known hypercortisolism, no systematic evaluation of its reliability in a consecutive series of patients with hypercortisolism has been published. Shortly after the introduction of this procedure, evidence was published showing that abnormal results were frequently seen in patients who had been hospitalized with pituitary tumors[11] or with other disorders[12] in the absence of Cushing's syndrome or evident stress. Recently the authors of this so-called overnight dexamethasone suppression test have reported a more serious deficiency in this procedure, viz., its failure to detect one of an unknown number of patients with Cushing's syndrome, apparently because of unusually slow turnover of the dexamethasone.[13] To obviate the possibility that retarded dexamethasone turnover might result in failure to recognize Cushing's

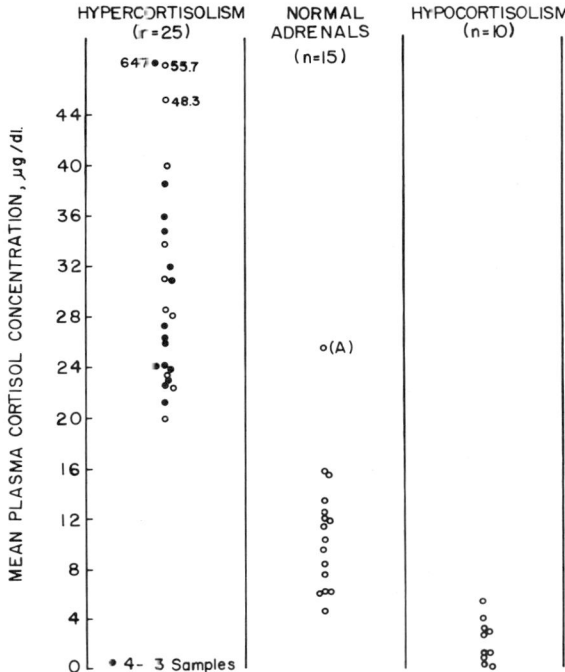

Fig. 5-2. Mean plasma cortisol concentration derived from 4–48 determinations evenly spaced throughout 24 hr in 25 patients with hypercortisolism, 15 subjects with normal adrenal function, and 10 patients with primary or secondary adrenal insufficiency. The normal range, 4.5–16 µg/dl (excluding one "normal" subject who was persistently and severely apprehensive), is clearly below the values found in any patient with hypercortisolism.

syndrome by the overnight suppression test, the authors suggest measurement of the plasma dexamethasone concentration simultaneously with the plasma cortisol determination at 8 A.M. Unfortunately, this necessity destroys the potential usefulness of this procedure as a simple screening test for Cushing's syndrome, since measurements of plasma dexamethasone concentrations are not available in many hospitals. A systematic study of the frequency of this shortcoming of the overnight dexamethasone suppression test is badly needed. Until such time as this has been done, it would seem rather dangerous to rely solely on this test for the diagnostic exclusion of Cushing's syndrome.

TWO-DAY DEXAMETHASONE TEST OF LIDDLE

In the procedure of Liddle,[14] urinary 17-OHCS excretion is measured on the second day of the administration of dexamethasone (0.5 mg every 6 hr). Cushing's syndrome is said to be characterized by urinary 17-OHCS excretion of more than 4.0 mg on the second day of dexamethasone administration. When it was introduced in 1960 this test constituted a very useful advance in the diagnosis of Cushing's syndrome. It was clearly superior to procedures being employed in many other centers in an attempt to find a consistently reliable method of distinguishing between patients with Cushing's syndrome and patients with normal adrenocortical function on the basis of differences in responses to adrenal

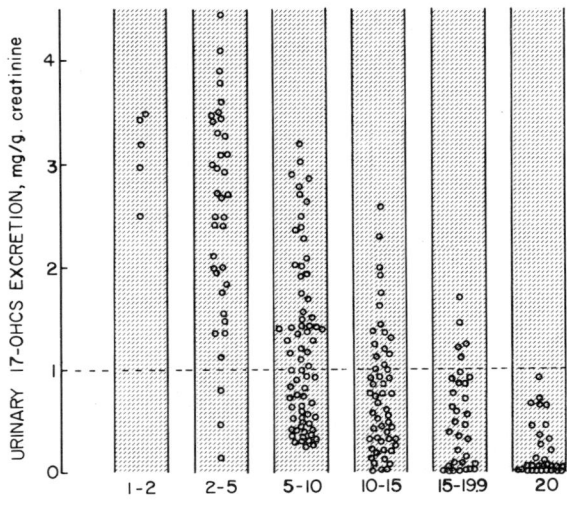

Fig. 5-3. Effects of increasing oral doses of dexamethasone on urinary excretion of 17-OHCS (per gram of urinary creatinine) in 32 normal subjects. Note that when the dose of dexamethasone was 20 μg/kg/day, or 5 μg/kg every 6 hr, urinary 17-OHCS excretion was invariably below 1 mg/g creatinine in the normal individuals.

suppression by administration of prednisone, fludrocortisone, and other exogenous steroids.[15,16] However, since its introduction steadily increasing numbers of instances have been reported in which this procedure failed to detect the presence of Cushing's syndrome in patients in whom the disorder could be unequivocally authenticated by other reliable criteria.[2,3,17-19] The frequency of these false negative results with Liddle's procedure will be discussed and compared with the results of other diagnostic tests below.

MODIFIED 2-DAY DEXAMETHASONE SUPPRESSION TEST

Streeten et al.[2] investigated the possibility that whereas the standard dose of dexamethasone proposed by Liddle[14] was appropriate for diagnosis of Cushing's syndrome in patients with obesity, it might be too large for recognition of hypercortisolism in smaller or less obese patients. Dose–response relationships were determined between various doses of dexamethasone and urinary excretion of 17-OHCS per gram of creatinine in lean and obese normal subjects. The results obtained from observations of 32 normal subjects are shown in Figure 5–3. The stepwise reduction in 17-OHCS excretion with increasing dosage of dexamethasone is clearly evident. When the dose of dexamethasone was 20 μg/kg/day or 5 μg/kg every 6 hr, urinary 17-OHCS fell below 1 mg/g creatinine in all 32 subjects. In contrast, urinary 17-OHCS excretion was suppressed below 1 mg/g creatinine in none of 21 patients with good collateral evidence of hypercortisolism.[2] Six of these 21 patients had fallaciously normal responses to the dexamethasone suppression procedure of Liddle,[14] an incidence of 29 percent false negative results. A further direct comparison of the reliabilities of the dexamethasone doses proposed by Liddle (0.5 mg every 6 hr) and those used by our group (5 μg/kg every 6 hr) in 29 patients with hypercortisolism is reported later in this chapter.

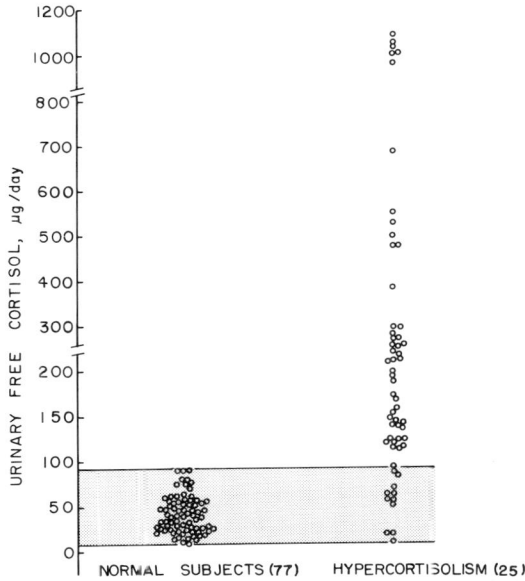

Fig. 5-4. Measurements of urinary free cortisol excretion in 77 normal subjects and 25 patients with hypercortisolism, most but not all of whose determinations were above the normal range (10–90 μg/day).

Urinary Excretion of Free Cortisol

Cope at al.[15,20] and Murphy[21] showed that urinary excretion of unmetabolized (free) cortisol was above normal limits in patients with hypercortisolism. Several authors have supported the usefulness of urinary free cortisol measurements in the diagnosis of hypercortisolism, but there have been no reports on the validity of the diagnostic conclusions reached on the basis of a comparison of these measurements with evidence derived from other observations. Figure 5–4 shows that the vast majority of measurements of urinary free cortisol in patients with undoubted hypercortisolism were well above the normal range. However, urinary free cortisol fell within the normal range in 11 determinations on these patients, with consistently "normal" results in 9 of 25 patients. Thus this measurement may be considered to provide strong confirmatory evidence of the presence of hypercortisolism, but it should be expected to give false negative results in approximately 36 percent of patients.

Cortisol Secretion Rate

The cortisol secretion rate is a research tool that still is not generally available for use in the diagnosis of hypercortisolism. When expressed in terms of urinary creatinine excretion,[2] the cortisol secretion rate is consistently elevated above the upper limit of the normal range (4–19 mg/g creatinine per day) in patients with hypercortisolism (Fig. 5–5).

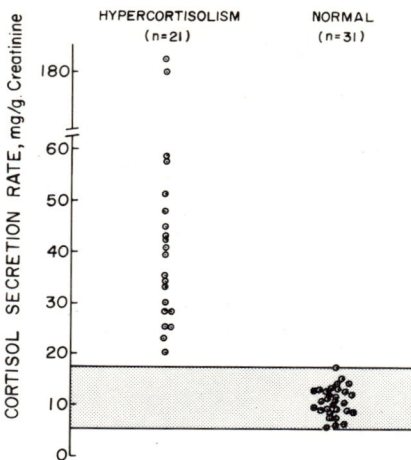

Fig. 5-5. Cortisol secretion rates (in milligrams per gram of urinary creatinine per day) in 21 patients with hypercortisolism; rates were all above the range of these determinations (4–19 mg/g creatinine per day) in 31 normal subjects.

Comparison of the Diagnostic Tests

Figure 5–6 provides a cortisol profile of patients in whom the clinical findings, most laboratory determinations, and the results of therapy conclusively indicated the presence of hypercortisolism. The figure compares the usefulness of the following tests: (1) the mean of 2 or 3 measurements of urinary 17-OHCS excretion per gram of creatinine; (2) the mean of 2 or 3 measurements of urinary free cortisol; (3) the mean of 4 to 48 determinations of plasma cortisol by the methods of Silber and Porter,[23] Mattingly,[24] or Murphy[21] (competitive protein binding) or by radioimmunoassay on plasma samples obtained at equal spacing throughout the day and night (every 30 min in 10 patients and every 2–6 hr in 15 patients); (4) urinary 17-OHCS excretion on the second day of dexamethasone at 0.5 mg every 6 hr (expressed as milligrams per day) and on the second day of dexamethasone at 5.0 μg/kg every 6 hr (expressed as milligrams per gram of creatinine per day); (5) cortisol secretion rate measured as described previously[2] (expressed as milligrams per gram of creatinine per day).

The crosshatched area in Figure 5–6 delineates the normal range, determined by measurements on between 24 and 150 subjects for each of the procedures. It is clear that there is complete agreement between the diagnostic conclusions from urinary 17-OHCS (per gram of creatinine), mean plasma cortisol concentration, urinary 17-OHCS (per gram of creatinine) during dexamethasone (5 μg/kg/6 hr), and cortisol secretion rates (per gram of creatinine) in all 29 patients with hypercortisolism. On the other hand, urinary free cortisol results failed to reveal the presence of hypercortisolism in 9 patients, while the Liddle test (dexamethasone 0.5 mg every 6 hr) gave false negative results in 8 patients, only 2 of whom were patients whose results of free cortisol excretion were discordant. It seems reasonable to conclude that urinary free cortisol measurements and the suppression test of Liddle are unreliable and should be replaced by the other four procedures listed.

Diagnosis and Treatment of Cushing's Syndrome

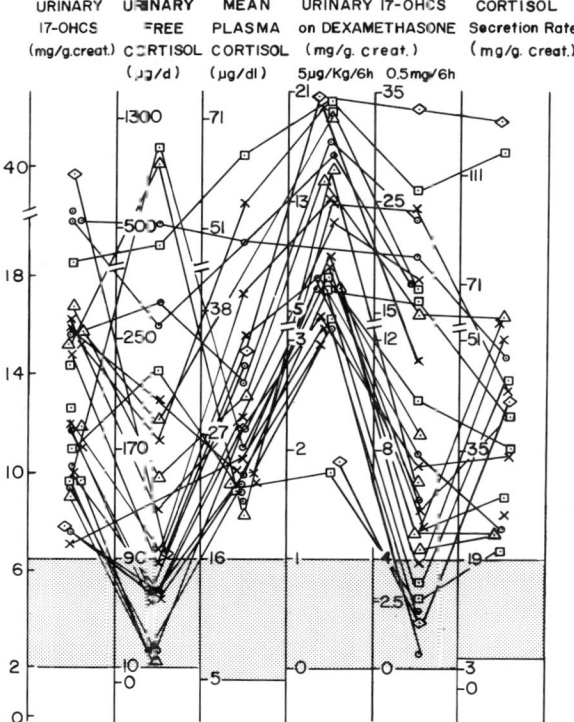

Fig. 5-6. Cortisol profile in 29 patients with hypercortisolism. There is complete separation between the results in normal subjects (stippled areas) and those in patients with hypercortisolism in urinary 17-OHCS (milligrams per gram of creatinine, mean of 2–3 24 hr urines), mean plasma cortisol concentration (4–48 determinations evenly spaced throughout 24 hr), urinary 17-OHCS (milligrams per gram of creatinine) on the second day of dexamethasone administration (5 μg/kg/6 hr), and cortisol secretion rate (milligrams per gram of urinary creatinine per day). In contrast, several of the patients with strong evidence of hypercortisolism had misleadingly "normal" results of urinary free cortisol and urinary 17-OHCS on the second day of dexamethasone (0.5 mg/6 hr).

PATHOLOGIC DIAGNOSIS OF HYPERCORTISOLISM

When the presence of hypercortisolism has been firmly established by the criteria described above, it is necessary to determine, if possible, whether the disorder results from adrenocortical adenoma, adrenocortical carcinoma, bilateral adrenocortical hyperplasia with or without pituitary adenoma or carcinoma, ectopic ACTH-producing neoplasm, or exogenous steroid or ACTH administration.

The large-dose dexamethasone suppression test of Liddle (2 mg every 6 hr for 2 days) is still the best method of differentiating between patients with adrenocortical steroid-producing and ectopic ACTH-producing tumors whose urinary 17-OHCS excretion is not significantly affected by dexamethasone (2 mg every 6 hr) and patients with bilateral adrenocortical hyperplasia, whose 17-OHCS excretion is almost invariably reduced by at least 50 percent on the second day of dexamethasone administration. Occasional instances have been encountered[25] (we have seen 3 cases) of patients with hypercortisolism of hypothalamic or pituitary origin in whom dexamethasone (2 mg every 6 hr) failed to reduce steroid excretion significantly. In 2 of these patients (both studied with the kind collaboration of Dr. A.M. Moses) the presence of pituitary carcinoma became evident many months after the excision of bilaterally hyperplastic adrenals. Occasional instances have also been reported of "normal" suppression of urinary 17-OHCS excretion by dexamethasone in patients with adrenal tumors.[25,27]

Other methods of differentiating tumors from bilateral hyperplasia of the adrenals are as follows:

1. Measurements of plasma ACTH are usually elevated in hypercortisolism of hypothalamic, pituitary, or ectopic origin[28] and suppressed in patients with adrenal tumors and in patients who are taking large doses of glucocorticoids.
2. Metyrapone (Metopirone) tests have been shown to produce exaggerated responses in most patients with hypercortisolism caused by bilateral adrenocortical hyperplasia and subnormal responses in patients with adrenocortical or ectopic tumors.[29] In our experience metyrapone usually (but by no means always) stimulates an exaggerated response in patients with bilateral adrenal hyperplasia and may be associated with a normal response in patients with adrenal tumors (Fig. 5–7). This test is not comparable in reliability to the large-dose dexamethasone suppression test.
3. An exaggerated response in urinary 17-OHCS excretion on the day of a standard 8-hr ACTH infusion (preferably done with 0.25 mg of cosyntropin, a synthetic α^{1-24}-corticotropin) is usually but not always seen in patients with bilateral adrenocortical hyperplasia (Fig. 5–7). This procedure is also unreliable.
4. Simultaneous bilateral adrenal vein and peripheral vein plasma cortisol determinations are useful in differentiating between adrenocortical neoplasms, which are invariably unilateral, and bilateral adrenocortical hyperplasia due to ACTH excess derived from pituitary or ectopic sources.
5. Urinary 17-ketosteroid excretion is usually high; it is often extremely elevated in patients with adrenocortical carinoma and is modestly elevated in patients with hypercortisolism originating in the hypothalamus, the pituitary, or an ectopic ACTH-producing tumor. On the other hand, urinary 17-ketosteroids are usually subnormal or normal in patients with adrenocortical adenoma and in patients who are taking excessive doses of glucocorticoids.
6. A skull x-ray should always be obtained in patients with hypercortisolism to determine whether sellar enlargement is present, which would suggest the presence of a pituitary tumor.

The results of these tests will define the underlying pathology in almost all patients with hypercortisolism, as shown in Table 5–2.

Recognition of self-administration of steroids or ACTH in excessive amounts may be extremely difficult, particularly in patients who have valid prescriptions for modest or replacement doses of these substances. We have seen several patients whose striking

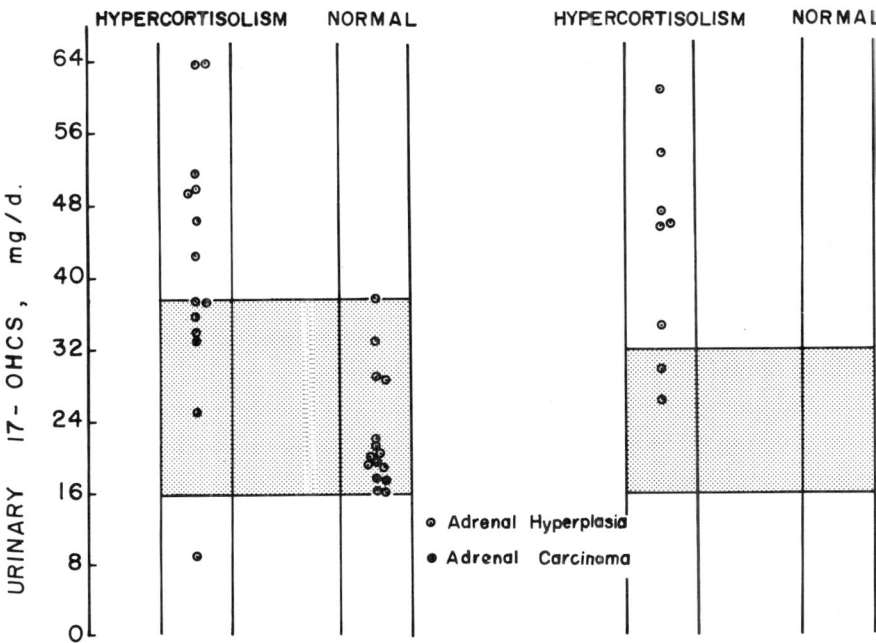

Fig. 5-7. Urinary 17-OHCS excretion on the day after metyrapone (500 mg every 2 hr for 12 doses) and on the day of ACTH (cosyntropin) infusion (0.25 mg over 8 hr) in patients with hypercortisolism and in normal subjects (stippled).

features of florid Cushing's syndrome seemed far in excess of the usual effects of prescribed maintenance doses of cortisol, but we have not encountered Cushing's syndrome caused by self-administration of ACTH. The diagnosis can usually be established by measuring urinary 17-OHCS output and plasma cortisol concentrations, both of which are usually high with excessive intake of cortisol and low with excessive intake of such steroids as dexamethasone. The results of dexamethasone suppression and other tests conducted during hospital admission would depend on the availability to the patient of a continuing supply of the steroid being taken and on the exact nature of the steroid ingested.

TREATMENT OF HYPERCORTISOLISM

Treatment of hypercortisolism depends on the cause of the disorder.

Adrenal adenomas should be excised after demonstration of their presence and location by means of adrenal vein cortisol determinations and adrenal phlebograms. Suppression of the contralateral adrenal by the tumor usually results in the need for steroid

Table 5-2
Methods of Differentiating Tumors and Bilateral Adrenal Hyperplasia

	Dexamethasone (2 mg every 6 hr) Suppression of Urinary 17-OHCS	Plasma ACTH	Adrenal Vein Cortisol	Metyrapone Test	ACTH Test	Urinary 17-Ketosteroids
Adrenocortical adenoma	Not reduced by > 50%	Low	High one side equals peripheral vein on other side	Poor response	Poor response	Low
Adrenocortical carcinoma	Not reduced by > 50%	Low	High one side equals peripheral vein on other side	Poor response	Poor response	High (often very high)
Hypothalmic disorder	Reduced by > 50%	High	High both sides	Exaggerated response	Exaggerated response	High
Pituitary tumor	Reduced by > 50%	High	High both sides	Exaggerated response	Exaggerated response	High
Ectopic tumor producing ACTH	Not reduced by > 50%	High (usually)	High both sides	Variable	Exaggerated response	High
Exogenous steroid Rx	Variable	Low	Low both sides	Poor response	Poor response	Low
Exogenous ACTH Rx	Not reduced by > 50%	High or variable	High both sides	Poor response	Exaggerated response	High

replacement therapy during and immediately after surgery,[30] with tapering of dosage when convalescence is complete and eventual discontinuation of all therapy.

Adrenal carcinomas should be removed without delay and treated with a course of irradiation therapy and steroid replacement therapy until contralateral adrenal regrowth has occurred. They may be treated with o,p'-DDD[31] with some improvement in the manifestations of Cushing's syndrome, but not always with noticeable change in size or rate of growth of the original or metastatic tumor.

Pituitary adenoma, when demonstrable, should be treated by irradiation therapy or by surgical resection using either the transsphenoidal route (for entirely intrasellar lesions) or open craniotomy (if extrasellar extension is present).

Hypothalamic and/or pituitary disease without demonstrable presence of pituitary tumor may be treated with any of a variety of methods, depending on available resources and on the patient's age, sex, and personal factors. When the disorder is relatively mild, and especially when it is encountered in an individual in the reproductive age group, pituitary irradiation is worthy of trial. If this is unsuccessful, as is often the case, bilateral total adrenalectomy is usually advisable. The 10–20 percent incidence of expanding chromophobe adenomas of the pituitary after bilateral adrenalectomy for Cushing's syndrome can probably be reduced by pituitary irradiation. Very severe hypercortisolism is best treated by bilateral adrenalectomy or hypophysectomy; if the hypercortisolism is associated with profound weakness, potassium depletion, or intractable psychic changes, it may be advisable to precede surgical therapy with a course of treatment with metyrapone (750 mg every 4 hr) or aminoglutethimide, together with replacement doses of dexamethasone (0.75 mg/day). In average cases of hypercortisolism, when the reproductive capacity of the individual does not need to be considered, hypophysectomy is probably the treatment of choice. Transsphenoidal resection is favored at present in our clinic, but implants of ^{90}Y seeds into the sella, cryosurgery of the pituitary, and proton-beam irradiation all have their advantages and disadvantages. Two forms of chemotherapy are at present undergoing trial. One of these, the administration of cyproheptadine (Periactin), is said to correct the hypothalamic disorder that is thought to cause Cushing's syndrome in the majority of cases.[32] The other, o,p'-DDD therapy, produces adrenal atrophy and is being used both for carcinoma and (experimentally) for bilateral adrenocortical hyperplasia.[31]

In hypercortisolism caused by ectopic ACTH-producing tumors, when the disorder is due to a solitary lesion such as a bronchial carcinoid tumor, a circumscribed bronchogenic carcinoma, a pancreatic carcinoma, or a tumor of the thymus, the practicability of surgical excision should be carefully considered, since great clinical improvement will frequently ensue. Even if no prolongation of life can be accomplished, relief of the symptoms of hypercortisolism will often improve the quality of life immeasurably.

Whichever form of therapy is used for the patient with Cushing's syndrome, it is important to be aware of the need for cortisol replacement therapy acutely and after the actual treatment. The patient, the spouse, or a close relative should be given a card describing the treatment performed and the need for increased steroid dosage in the event of stresses supervening in the future[30]

Patients and their relatives can be reassured that gradual, steady, and often remarkable improvement in all features of hypercortisolism (except for the features of vascular damage) is to be expected within 2 to 8 months of surgical therapy. Absence of such improvement usually implies a wrong diagnosis in the first place, or such unusual occurrences as growth of accessory adrenal glands or excessive self-medication.

REFERENCES

1. Cushing H: The basophil adenomas of the pituitary body and their clinical manifestations (pituitary basophilism). Bull Johns Hopkins Hosp 50:137, 1932
2. Streeten DHP, Stevenson CT, Dalakos TG, et al: The diagnosis of hypercortisolism. Biochemical criteria differentiating patients from lean and obese normal subjects and from females on oral contraceptives. J Clin Endocrinol Metab 29:1191, 1969
3. Schletter FE, Clift GV, Meyer R, et al: Cushing's syndrome in childhood: Report of two cases with bilateral adrenocortical hyperplasia, showing distinctive features. J Clin Endocrinol Metab 27:22, 1967
4. Streeten DHP, Faas FH, Elders MJ, et al: Hypercortisolism in childhood. Shortcomings of conventional diagnostic criteria. Pediatrics 56:797, 1975
5. Nugent CA, Nichols T, Tyler FH: Diagnosis of Cushing's syndrome. Single dose dexamethasone suppression test. Arch Intern Med 116:172, 1965
6. Pavlatos FC, Smilo RP, Forsham PH: A rapid screening test for Cushing's syndrome. JAMA 193:720, 1965
7. Krieger DT, Allen W, Rizzo F, et al: Characterization of the normal temporal pattern of plasma corticosteroid levels. J Clin Endocrinol Metab 32:266, 1971
8. Hellman L, Nakada F, Curti J, et al: Cortisol is secreted episodically. J Clin Endocrinol Metab 30:411, 1970
9. Tourniaire J, Orgiazzi J, Riviere JF, et al: Repeated plasma cortisol determinations in Cushing's syndrome due to adrenocortical adenoma. J Clin Endocrinol Metab 22:666, 1971
10. Sederberg-Olsen P, Binder C, Kehlet H, et al: Episodic variation in plasma corticosteroids in subjects with Cushing's syndrome of differing etiology. J Clin Endocrinol Metab 36:906, 1973
11. Moses AM, Miller M: Stimulation and inhibition of ACTH release in patients with pituitary disease. J Clin Endocrinol Metab 28:1581, 1968
12. Connolly CK, Gore MBR, Stanley N, et al: Single dose dexamethasone suppression in normal subjects and hospital patients. Br Med J 2:665, 1968
13. Meikle AW, Lagerquist LG, Tyler FH: Apparently normal pituitary-adrenal suppressibility in Cushing's syndrome: Dexamethasone metabolism and plasma levels. J Lab Clin Med 86:472, 1975
14. Liddle GW: Tests of pituitary-adrenal suppressibility in the diagnosis of Cushing's syndrome. J Clin Endocrinol Metab 20:1539, 1960
15. Cope CL, Black EG: The reliability of some adrenal function tests. Br Med J 2:1117, 1959
16. Cope CL: Diagnostic use of adrenal inhibition in Cushing's syndrome. Br Med J 2:193, 1956
17. Schteingart DE, Gregerman RI, Conn JW: A comparison of the characteristics of increased adrenocortical function in obesity and in Cushing's syndrome. Metabolism 12:484, 1963
18. Braverman LE, Woeber KA, Ingbar SH: An unusual case of Cushing's syndrome. N Engl J Med 273:1018, 1965
19. Cassidy CE, Rosenfeld PS, Bokat MA: Suppression of activity of the adrenal cortex by dexamethasone in Cushing's syndrome. J Clin Endocrinol Metab 26:1181, 1966
20. Cope CL, Black E: The production rate of cortisol in man. Br Med J 1:1020, 1958
21. Murphy BEP: Clinical evaluation of urinary cortisol determinations by competitive protein-binding radioassay. J Clin Endocrinol Metab 28:343, 1968
22. Cope CL: The adrenal cortex in internal medicine — Part I. Br Med J 2:847, 1966
23. Silber RH, Porter CC: The determination of 17,21-dihydroxy-20-ketosteroids in urine and plasma. J Biol Chem 210:923, 1954
24. Mattingly D: A simple fluorimetric method for the estimation of free 11-hydroxycorticoids in human plasma. J Clin Pathol 15:374, 1962
25. Meador CK, Bowdoin B, Owen WC Jr, et al: Primary adrenocortical nodular dysplasia. A rare cause of Cushing's syndrome. J Clin Endocrinol Metab 27:1255, 1967
26. Silverman SR, Marnell RT, Sholiton LJ, et al: Failure of dexamethasone suppression test to indicate bilateral adrenocortical hyperplasia in Cushing's syndrome. J Clin Endocrinol Metab 23:167, 1963
27. Kendall JW, Sloop PR Jr: Dexamethasone-suppressible adrenocortical tumor. N Engl J Med 279:532, 1968
28. Liddle GW, Nicholson WE, Island DP, et al: Clinical and laboratory studies of ectopic humoral syndromes. Recent Prog Horm Res 25:283, 1969
29. Weiss ER, Rayyis SS, Nelson DH, et al: Evaluation of stimulation and suppression tests in the etiological diagnosis of Cushing's syndrome. Ann Intern Med 71:941, 1969
30. Streeten DHP: Corticosteroid therapy II. Complications and therapeutic indications. JAMA 232:1046, 1975

31. Temple TE, Jones DJ, Liddle GW, et al: Treatment of Cushing's disease. Correction of hypercortisolism by *o,p'*DDD without induction of aldosterone deficiency. N Engl J Med 281:801, 1969

32. Krieger DT, Amorosa L, Linick F: Cyproheptadine-induced remission of Cushing's disease. N Engl J Med 293:893, 1975

Gordon H. Williams

6
Renin-Angiotensin-Aldosterone Axis and Hypertension

Over the past few decades extensive evaluations of the renin-angiotensin-aldosterone axis have been performed, particularly in reference to individuals with elevated blood pressure. The rationale for these investigations is apparent when one considers that volume and peripheral resistance are the major components involved in blood pressure control, since the renin-angiotensin system plays a unique role in the regulation of both of these components. The purpose of this chapter is to update information on the regulation of this system and to point out several areas in which abnormalities in its regulation may play a significant role in the pathophysiology of the hypertensive process.

PHYSIOLOGY OF THE RENIN-ANGIOTENSIN-ALDOSTERONE SYSTEM

Although a number of adrenal steroids promote sodium retention and potassium loss, aldosterone is the major mineralocorticoid produced by the adrenal cortex. Under normal circumstances aldosterone has two important physiologic functions: it has an important role in the regulation of extracellular fluid volume, and it is a major determinant of potassium metabolism. Aldosterone acts at the distal convoluted tubule of the kidney to promote sodium reabsorption and to increase urinary excretion of potassium. The absorption of sodium from the filtrate is active (i.e., it requires energy expenditure), while potassium apparently flows passively to neutralize the electrochemical gradient. Hydrogen ions may also be lost in the urine by the same mechanism. Thus, in order for urinary potassium wasting and hypokalemia to occur, both an excess of aldosterone and sufficient sodium at the distal tubule exchange site are required.

There are three well-identified control mechanisms for aldosterone release: the renin-angiotensin system, potassium, and ACTH. Although a number of studies have demonstrated that ACTH stimulates aldosterone secretion, it seems to be less important than potassium and the renin-angiotensin system in the control of aldosterone production.

On the other hand, the renin-angiotensin system and potassium may be of equal importance in the regulation of aldosterone secretion.[1]

The renin-angiotensin system is a major system for the control of extracellular fluid volume through its regulation of aldosterone secretion. The renin-angiotensin system maintains the circulating blood volume by causing aldosterone-induced sodium retention during periods registered as volume deficiencies and by decreasing aldosterone secretion under conditions when volume is normal. The enzyme renin is secreted by the juxtaglomerular apparatus of the kidney and is released in response to a decrease in effective blood volume. Renin then acts on a circulating protein, angiotensinogen, to split off angiotensin I, which is rapidly acted on by converting enzymes located primarily in the lung to form angiotensin II, a potent vasoconstrictor and aldosterone-stimulating hormone. Increased aldosterone secretion will produce sodium retention and repair the volume deficit.

A number of recent studies have suggested that the response of this system to acute changes in volume is both rapid and sensitive. In one study the levels of plasma renin activity, angiotensin II, and aldosterone decreased by as much as 50 percent within the first hour of infusing normal saline at a rate of 500 ml/hr into normal sodium-restricted subjects.[2] This system is equally responsive to stimuli that produce volume depletion. It has been shown that within 5 min of assuming the upright position, renin levels are significantly elevated in normal subjects.[3]

In addition to its major effect on sodium homeostasis through its action on aldosterone secretion, angiotensin II is the most potent vasoconstrictor agent endogenously produced in man. Thus it can play a significant role in maintaining normal blood pressure, and it can obviously produce hypertension.

The adrenal glomerulosa and vascular smooth-muscle cells respond to similar angiotensin II levels. Thus, recent studies comparing the responses of vascular and adrenal tissue to angiotensin II have demonstrated a significant effect of sodium intake on these responses.[4] Graded infusions of angiotensin II in normal subjects on high-sodium intake produced much greater increments in blood pressure than in subjects on sodium-restricted intake. On the other hand, aldosterone responses on the sodium-restricted intake were greater than in the sodium-loaded state. Thus sodium intake reciprocally influences vascular and adrenal responses to angiotensin II. Salt restriction blunts the vascular response and potentiates the adrenal response—a physiologically important influence in view of aldosterone's role in sodium conservation. Furthermore, derangement in this relationship potentially could lead to elevated blood pressure.

The potassium ion can regulate aldosterone secretion independently of the renin-angiotensin system. Increasing the oral intake or blood levels of potassium will cause an increase in aldosterone secretion. This is an exquisitely sensitive mechanism, since significant increments in aldosterone levels have been shown to occur with changes in serum potassium of less than 0.2 mEq/liter. Potassium and aldosterone are involved in a negative-feedback loop system: following an increase in serum potassium, total body potassium, and/or intracellular potassium there is an increase in aldosterone secretion, which produces an increase in potassium excretion, thereby dampening out the initial stimulus for the increased aldosterone secretion. Thus, under ordinary circumstances, potassium and the renin-angiotensin system are probably of equal importance, with the level of aldosterone secreted being determined by the integration of signals from each negative-feedback loop (Fig. 6–1). Therefore the estimation of aldosterone secretion must be interpreted in light of these various regulatory factors.

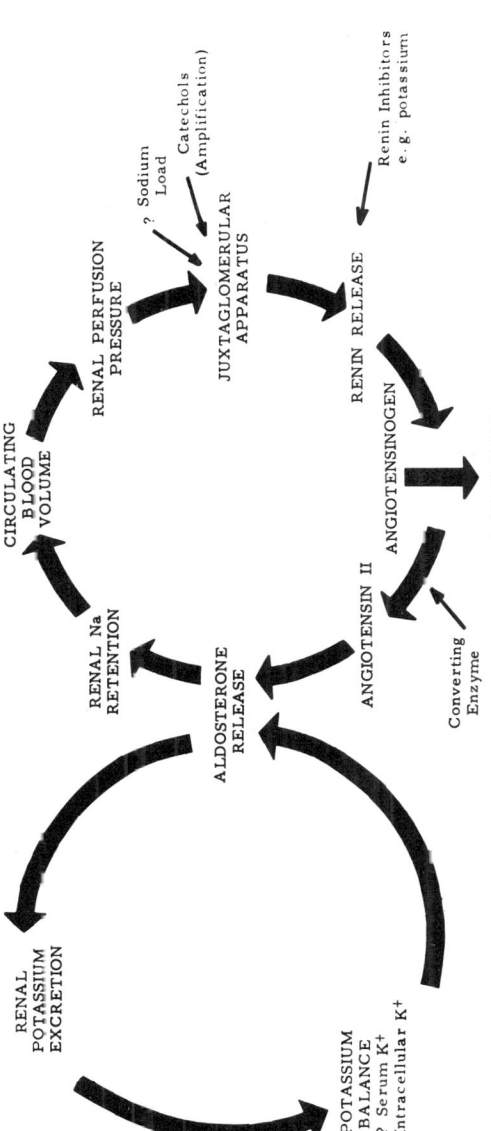

Fig. 6–1. Interrelationship of the volume and potassium feedback loops in aldosterone secretion. Integration of signals from each loop determines the level of aldosterone secreted. (Reproduced by permission from Williams GH, Dluhy RG: Aldosterone biosynthesis: Interrelationship of regulatory factors. Am J Med 53:595, 1972.)

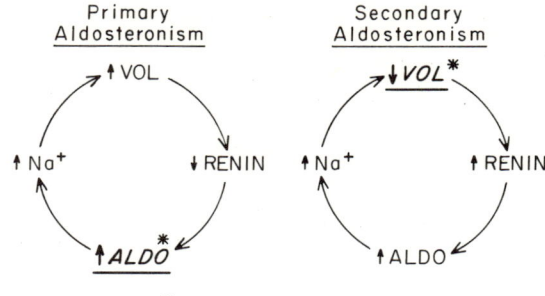

Fig. 6–2. Responses of the renin-aldosterone volume control loop in primary versus secondary aldosteronism. (Reproduced by permission from Williams GH, Dluhy RG, Thorn GW: Diseases of the adrenal cortex, in: Harrison's Principles of Internal Medicine (ed 7). 1974, p 508.)

HYPERTENSION AND HYPERALDOSTERONISM

Hyperaldosteronism may be present in hypertensive patients for either of two reasons (Fig. 6–2). Probably the most common cause is secondary to increased activity of the renin-angiotensin system (secondary aldosteronism). The increase in renin activity is usually secondary to a decrease in renal blood flow and/or perfusion pressure. This could be the result of narrowing of one or both major renal arteries by an atherosclerotic plaque or fibromuscular hyperplasia. Alternatively, it may be caused by profound vasoconstriction (accelerated phase of hypertension) or severe arteriolar fibrinoid necrosis (malignant hypertension). Patients with secondary aldosteronism exhibit the characteristic features of hyperaldosteronism, i.e., hypokalemic alkalosis and moderate to marked increases in aldosterone levels. However, in contrast to patients with primary aldosteronism, they have increased levels of renin activity.

The second cause of hyperaldosteronism is the result of primary overproduction of aldosterone by the adrenal gland. Most cases are secondary to small solitary adenomas. In a number of recent reports this syndrome has also been linked with bilateral adrenal cortical hyperplasia. Furthermore, it is now recognized that cases may present without the classic clinical and chemical features, thus obscuring the diagnosis. Renin activity in patients with primary aldosteronism is characteristically low.[5]

LOW-RENIN HYPERTENSION

The most frequently evaluated component in the renin-angiotensin-aldosterone axis in patients with hypertension is the plasma renin response to acute stimulation. In 1965 Helmer reported that 29 percent of 600 patients with hypertension had values less than normotensive controls under basal conditions.[6] Since that time there have been numerous reports assessing renin responsiveness in patients with hypertension. Most of these reports have defined a category variously termed low-renin hypertension or hyporesponsive renin essential hypertension, although it is also apparent that some patients with hypertension have increased renin release in response to acute stimulation.

A number of stimuli have been used to define the low-renin state. In most studies plasma renin activity has been assessed, although in a few cases plasma renin concentration has been used. There have been no apparent discrepancies between these methods, although comparative data are still meager. The majority of studies have used a low sodium intake and upright posture to define renin responsiveness. However, this requires hospitalization and rigorous dietary control—a procedure impractical for mass screening of large groups of hypertensive patients. Thus two outpatient procedures have been developed in recent years. The first is the renin response to acute administration of a potent diuretic, such as furosemide. One variant of this test assesses the renin response 30–90 min after intravenous administration of furosemide, a modification of the procedure originally used by Rosenthal et al. in normal subjects.[7] A second variant is to give oral furosemide, either in divided doses over a 12-hr period or as a single dose, and assess the renin response to upright posture 4 hr later.[8] A second outpatient procedure is to correlate 24-hr urine sodium excretion and upright plasma renin activity. A nomogram can then be developed between the amount of sodium excreted and plasma renin activity. This nomogram can be used to assess whether plasma renin activity is normal, high, or subnormal on any given sodium intake.[9]

Despite the wide variety of procedures to stimulate plasma renin activity, there is a remarkably consistent incidence of patients with low or hyporesponsive renin activity. This incidence ranges between 20 and 35 percent if patients with mineralocorticoid excess are excluded. It is also clear that separation of the low-renin group is easier if the patients have undergone some form of volume depletion as well as upright activity prior to sampling. In addition, a number of other variables have also been proposed as influencing the responsiveness of renin activity in both normal and hypertensive patients.

In some studies age, sex, race, diastolic blood pressure, duration of hypertension, and aldosterone secretory-excretory rates have been correlated with renin responsiveness. Nearly all studies in which a significant number of hypertensive subjects have been reported have indicated that those in the low-renin subgroup are significantly older than those in the normal-renin subgroup. In the more than 500 patients in the literature in which renin responsiveness and age have been correlated, the mean age for the low-renin subgroup is 47.1 years, while the mean age for the normal-renin subgroup is 39.5 years.[10]

No study has found a correlation between the duration of hypertension and the incidence of low-renin essential hypertension. This lack of correlation between age and duration in the incidence of low-renin hypertension may reflect our inability to determine precisely the onset of hypertension in these patients, since most are probably asymptomatic for variable periods of time before elevated blood pressure is documented.

A few studies have reported an increased incidence of low-renin hypertension in women with hypertension, while others have reported a higher incidence of low-renin hypertension in black subjects. The latter observation has recently been clarified, since normotensive black subjects have lower levels of plasma renin activity than white subjects. Thus, in defining the incidence of low renin activity in the black population, a pool of black normotensive subjects is necessary.

Finally, Schalekamp and his colleagues have suggested that renin release may be suppressed in hypertensive patients because of the increased intravascular pressure at the level of the juxtaglomerular cell.[11] This postulation would predict that those individuals with higher blood pressures would have lower levels of renin activity. Most studies, however, have not found a simple correlation between renin responsiveness and the level of blood pressure, although several have suggested that low-renin hypertensive subjects tend to have higher mean diastolic blood pressure levels than normal-renin subjects.

Intensive investigations over the last several years have been directed at uncovering

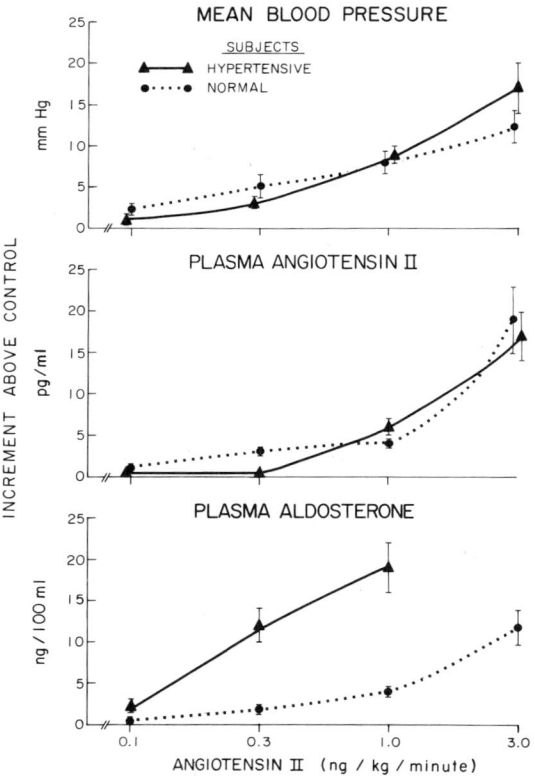

Fig. 6-3. Increments in plasma angiotensin II, plasma aldosterone, and mean blood pressure in response to graded infusions of angiotensin II in 7 normotensive and 12 hypertensive subjects (mean ± SEM). All subjects were studied supine, in balance, on a 200 mEq sodium/100 mEq potassium intake. There were no significant differences in the plasma angiotensin II concentrations. Threshold sensitivities for blood pressure were similar (between 0.3 and 1 ng/kg/min) in the groups; however, the increment in blood pressure at 3 ng/kg/min was significantly greater ($p < 0.05$) in the hypertensive group. On the other hand, both threshold sensitivity and peak response for aldosterone secretion were significantly greater in the hypertensive group ($p < 0.01$). (Reproduced by permission from Kisch ES, Dluhy RG, Williams GH: Enhanced aldosterone response to angiotensin II in human hypertension. Circ Res 38:502, 1976.)

the mechanism for the low-renin state. Most studies have examined the possibility of volume expansion producing the low renin, presumably secondary to another aldosteronelike mineralocorticoid. Several steroids, such as 18-hydroxydesoxycorticosterone, have been proposed as the agents producing the low-renin state.[12,13] However, there is no conclusive evidence that patients with low renin activity are necessarily volume-expanded. Direct measurements of exchangeable sodium in several recent studies have not supported earlier reports that individuals with low renin activity have expanded blood or extracellular fluid volumes.[14-17]

Renin-Angiotensin-Aldosterone Axis and Hypertension

The most intriguing recent suggestion has been that the suppressed renin levels are due to a change in the adrenal's sensitivity to angiotensin II. This hypothesis is an extension of the reports mentioned earlier in this chapter relative to the change in adrenal sensitivity induced in normal subjects with sodium restriction. Thus, perhaps some individuals with hypertension have enhanced adrenal reponse to angiotensin II. The volume renin-aldosterone feedback loop could then be closed with lower levels of angiotensin II, an appropriate adaptive mechanism in a subject with an elevated blood pressure. Supporting this hypothesis is a recent study reporting that patients with hypertension on high-sodium intake do have enhanced adrenal response to angiotensin II, as compared to normotensive individuals[18] (Fig. 6-3).

SCREENING PROCEDURES FOR PRIMARY ALDOSTERONISM

Of the 20 to 30 million individuals in the United States who are hypertensive, only a small fraction (0.1-2 percent) have primary aldosteronism. In addition, confirmation of the diagnosis of primary aldosteronism involves a series of complex and costly maneuvers. Thus the dilemma facing the physician is how to screen for this potentially curable form of hypertension that affects only a small fraction of the total hypertensive population.

It has been the experience of a number of investigators that screening patients for primary aldosteronism can be effectively accomplished by using serum potassium determinations. Except under unusual circumstances, this study can be performed as part of a routine office or outpatient evaluation. Individuals who have a positive response to these screening procedures should then be referred to a medical center that is equipped to carry out the complex procedures to confirm the diagnosis and determine whether the hyperaldosteronism is caused by an adenoma or bilateral hyperplasia[19] (Fig. 6-4).

If serum potassium level is used as the initial screening procedure, normal serum potassium levels exclude primary aldosteronism except under three specific circumstances. Serum potassium levels may be normal in patients with primary aldosteronism if they have been on a severe sodium-restricted intake, thus minimizing the loss of potassium from the distal tubule in the presence of excess aldosterone. Normokalemia may also be seen in individuals who have markedly increased their potassium intake (usually greater than 200 mEq/day) or in patients treated with an aldosterone antagonist (spironolactone or triamterene).

An effective screening test is to discontinue all diuretic therapy, place the patient on 10 g (170 mEq) of sodium chloride per day for 3 days, and then repeat the serum potassium determination. If the serum potassium is again normal, it is unlikely that the patient has mineralocorticoid excess. If the serum potassium falls following sodium chloride ingestion, it is likely that the patient has hyperaldosteronism that fails to suppress, and referral should be made to an appropriate center for definitive evaluation. However, caution must be observed in using sodium chloride to provoke hypokalemia. If there is evidence of incipient or actual cardiac failure, or if blood pressure is excessively elevated, sodium chloride loading should not be given. It should also not be administered to hypokalemic patients, since in the presence of hyperaldosteronism the challenge of additional salt may further decrease potassium to dangerously low levels.

If the original serum potassium is low, there are three possible causes: primary aldosteronism, secondary aldosteronism, or diuretic-induced hypokalemia. If the hypokalemia is secondary to diuretic (thiazide) therapy, serum potassium should return to normal levels if medication is withheld for 10-14 days; if hypokalemia persists, the most

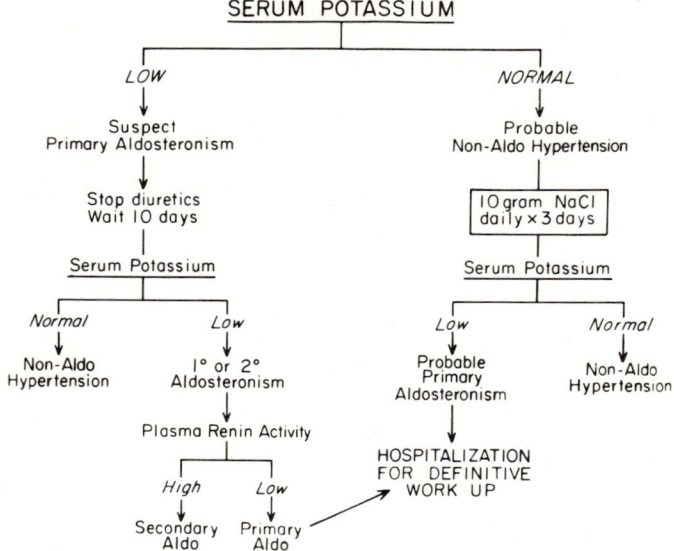

Fig. 6-4. Flow sheet for office screening of hypertensive patients for hyperaldosteronism. This is a summary of the material in the text. [Reproduced by permission from Williams GH, Dluhy RG: How to evaluate and manage hypokalemic high blood pressure, in Wolf GL, Eliot RS (eds): Practical Management of Hypertension. New York, Futura Publishing, 1975, p 47.]

likely diagnosis is hyperaldosteronism. Under these circumstances, obtaining a plasma renin activity in the morning, after the patient has been ambulatory for 1.5–2 hr, should differentiate between secondary and primary aldosteronism. In primary aldosteronism the value will be low, while in secondary aldosteronism the value will be high.

Patients who have positive responses to the screening procedure should then be referred to a specialized center equipped to carry out the complex and intricate diagnostic procedures necessary to confirm the diagnosis of primary aldosteronism and to determine the appropriate type of therapy to be used.

REFERENCES

1. Williams GH, Dluhy RG: Aldosterone biosynthesis: Interrelationship of regulatory factors. Am J Med 53:595, 1972
2. Tuck ML, Dluhy RG, Williams GH: A specific role for saline or the sodium ion in the regulation of renin and aldosterone secretion. J Clin Invest 53:988, 1974
3. Tuck ML, Dluhy RG, Williams GH: Sequential responses of the renin-angiotensin-aldosterone axis to acute postural change: Effect of dietary sodium. J Lab Clin Med 86:754, 1975
4. Hollenberg NK, Chenitz WR, Adams DF, et al: Reciprocal influence of salt intake on adrenal glomerulosa and renal vascular responses to angiotensin II in normal man. J Clin Invest 54:34, 1974
5. Williams GH, Dluhy RG: How to evaluate and manage hypokalemic high blood pressure, in Wolf GL, Eliot RS (eds): Practical Management of Hypertension. New York, Futura Publishing, 1975, pp 41–52
6. Helmer OM: The renin-angiotensin system and its relation to hypertension. Prog Cardiovasc Dis 8:117, 1965
7. Rosenthal J, Boucher R, Nowaczynski W, et al: Acute changes in plasma volume, renin activity, and free aldosterone levels in healthy subjects following furosemide administration. Can J Physiol Pharmacol 46:85, 1968
8. Carey RM, Douglas JG, Schweikert JR, et al: The syndrome of essential hypertension and suppressed plasma renin activity. Normalization

of blood pressure with spironolactone. Arch Intern Med 130:849, 1972
9. Brunner HR, Laragh JH, Baer L, et al: Essential hypertension: Renin and aldosterone, heart attack and stroke. N Engl J Med 286:441, 1972
10. Tuck ML, Williams GH, Cain JF, et al: Relation of age, diastolic pressure and known duration of hypertension to presence of low renin essential hypertension. Am J Cardiol 22:637, 1973
11. Schalekamp MADH, Krauss XH, Schalekamp-Kuyken MPA, et al: Studies on the mechanism of hyper-natriuresis in essential hypertension in relation to measurements of plasma renin concentration, body fluid compartments and renal function. Clin Sci 41:219, 1971
12. Melby JC, Dale SL, Wilson TE: 18-hydroxydeoxycorticosterone in human hypertension. Circ Res 28:143, 1971
13. Williams GH, Braley LM, Underwood RH: The regulation of plasma 18-hydroxy 11-deoxycorticosterone in man. J Clin Invest 58:221, 1976
14. Jose A, Crout JR, Kaplan NM: Suppressed plasma renin activity in essential hypertension. Ann Intern Med 72:9, 1970
15. Woods JW, Liddle GW, Stant EG Jr, et al: Effect of an adrenal inhibitor in hypertensive patients with suppressed renin. Ann Intern Med 123:366, 1969
16. Schalekamp MA, Lebel M, Beevers DG, et al: Body-fluid volume in low-renin hypertension. Lancet 2 310, 1974
17. Lebel M, Schalekamp MA, Beevers DG, et al: Sodium and the renin-angiotensin system in essential hypertension and mineralocorticoid excess. Lancet 2:308, 1974
18. Kisch ES, Dluhy RG, Williams GH: Enhanced aldosterone response to angiotensin II in human hypertension. Circ Res 38:502, 1976
19. Baer L, Sommers SC, Krakoff LR, et al: Pseudo-primary aldosteronism: An entity distinct from true primary aldosteronism. Circ Res 26,27[Suppl 1]:203, 1970

Paul G. Cohen

7
An Approach to the Hypertensive Patient

In recent years, greater understanding of the mechanisms and consequences of hypertension has led to a more vigorous approach to the screening, diagnosis, and treatment of this disease. Nevertheless, there is still great variability in the basic clinical evaluation of the hypertensive patient, among physicians and investigators alike.

The recognition that effective treatment has resulted in striking decreases in mortality and morbidity among hypertensive patients has placed new emphasis on diagnosis of curable forms of hypertension as well as on treatment of hypertension.[1,2] Furthermore, a large body of information has been accumulated about the pathogenesis and maintenance of a variety of hypertensive states. Great emphasis has been placed on the role of the renin-angiotensin-aldosterone system in the diagnosis of hypertension,[3-7] and Dr. Gordon Williams earlier reviewed the physiology in this area in detail. Alterations in this finely tuned homeostatic system may be either primary (i.e., Conn's syndrome or renin-secreting tumor) or secondary (excess salt intake) and should result in appropriate changes in the hormonal feedback loops. These physiologic changes can be categorized into a variety of patterns that help to screen for the curable causes of hypertension.

The current discussion will attempt to present a unified approach to physiologic evaluation of the hypertensive patient, utilizing commonly available outpatient resources. A relatively simple format is proposed, employing four common physiologic parameters that serve as discriminants for classifying many of the different forms of hypertension. These are a 24-hr urine determination of sodium and potassium, as well as determinations of plasma renin activity and serum potassium.

Figure 7–1 summarizes many of the possible interrelationships utilizing these four discriminants. After a diagnosis of hypertension is established, a 24-hr urine for sodium and potassium determinations is obtained, and determinations of plasma renin activity and serum potassium are made. Patients who excrete excessive salt are then placed on salt restriction. If their blood pressures are restored to normal, they are checked periodically. The patients who remain hypertensive are rechecked for reliability of salt restriction. If the salt intake is in fact reduced, then they are studied in a manner similar to other patients with sodium excretions in the normal range.

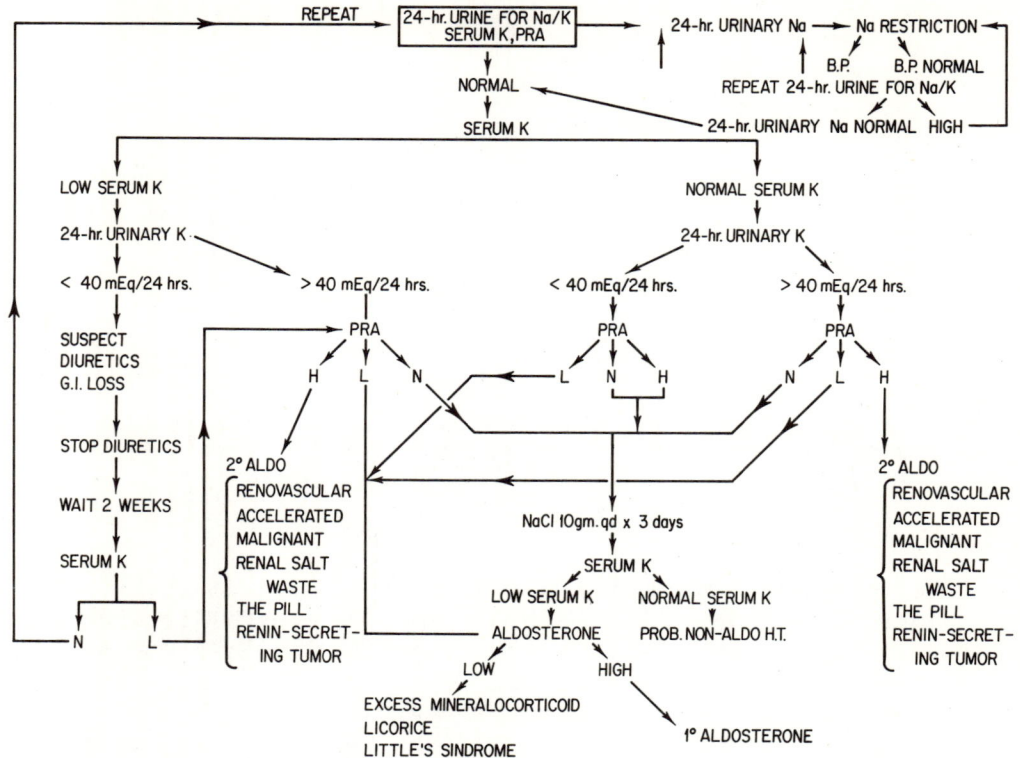

Fig. 7-1. Physiologic approach to hypertension.

SERUM AND URINARY POTASSIUM

The patients are divided on the basis of serum potassium into normal and low groups. Hypokalemia has been recognized as an important discriminant for primary aldosteronism. Several studies suggest that potassium levels below 3.6 mEq/liter should be further evaluated to establish the diagnosis of primary aldosteronism.[8,9]

The diagnostic specificity of serum potassium can be further sharpened by evaluation of 24-hr urinary excretion of potassium. The value of the urinary potassium determination is that it reflects distal tubular function and is modulated by both sodium excretion and aldosterone secretion. High urinary potassium excretion may occur with increased sodium intake; however, it is usually more indicative of the degree of adrenal aldosterone production.[8,9] It has been observed that most patients with primary aldosteronism excrete more than 40 mEq of potassium per 24 hr.[8] Therefore urinary potassium excretion of more than 40 mEq/24 hr, particularly in the presence of a low potassium level, is indicative of increased aldosterone secretion. This may occur with either the primary (Conn's syndrome) or secondary (renovascular hypertension) form of aldosteronism.

PLASMA RENIN ACTIVITY AND ALDOSTERONE

Plasma renin activity (PRA) can be utilized to further differentiate the nature of the presumed aldosterone state. A low PRA would be indicative of increased extracellular volume expansion, whereas a high PRA might indicate that the stimulus for PRA has been sensed (i.e., because of volume depletion). Classically, a patient profile of low serum potassium, increased urinary potassium, and low PRA is related to increased salt-retaining hormone production. This could be aldosterone or another salt-retaining hormone or substance (licorice). To differentiate these, a determination of plasma aldosterone level or excretion would be necessary. An increased aldosterone level would establish the diagnosis of primary aldosteronism.

There are some rare patients who have the low-renin profile and the appearance of primary aldosteronism but who have low aldosterone levels. Identified causes include excess nonaldosterone mineralocorticoid production, large amounts of licorice ingestion, and Little's syndrome.

SODIUM LOADING TEST

The administration of a sodium load results in an increased amount of sodium reaching the distal tubule. In the presence of an aldosterone state, or excess mineralocorticoid effect, there is a marked enhancement of potassium exchange, with resultant potassium excretion. In patients with normal serum potassium and predominantly normal PRA in whom an aldosterone state is suspected (i.e., increased urinary potassium excretion), sodium loading may unmask the hypokalemia. This can be helpful in detecting occult aldosteronism and differentiating it from nonaldosterone forms of hypertension.

REFERENCES

1. Freis E: Effects of treatment on morbidity in hypertension. Report of Veterans Administration cooperative study. JAMA 202:1028–1034, 1967
2. Freis E: Effects of treatment on morbidity in hypertension. Report of Veterans Administration cooperative study. JAMA 213:1143–1152, 1970
3. Laragh JH, Baer L, Brunner HR, et al: Renin, angiotensin and aldosterone system in pathogenesis and management of hypertensive vascular disease. Am J Med 52:633–652, 1972
4. Hollenberg NK, Epstein M, Basch RI, et al: Renin secretion in essential and accelerated hypertension. Am J Med 47:855–859, 1969
5. Saruta T, Saade GA, Kaplan NM: A possible mechanism for hypertension induced by oral contraceptives. Arch Intern Med 126:621–626, 1967
6. Bath NM, Gennells JC, Robinson RR: Plasma renin activity in renovascular hypertension. Am J Med 45:381–390, 1968
7. Williams GE, Rose LI, Dluhy RG, et al: Abnormal responsiveness of renin aldosterone system to acute stimulation in patients with essential hypertension. Ann Intern Med 72:317–326, 1970
8. Kaplan NM: Hypokalemia in the hypertensive patient. Ann Intern Med 66:1079–1090, 1967
9. Brown JJ, Davies DC, Fraser R, et al: Plasma electrolytes, renin, and aldosteronism in the diagnosis of primary hyperaldosteronism. Lancet 1:1028–1034, 1968

Leslie I. Rose

8
Evaluation and Therapy of the Hirsute Female

Hirsutism is a widespread problem in the United States, as witnessed by the large number of successful electrolysis centers in our major cities. For many individuals electrology is a reasonable answer; however, some women have hirsutism as a physical sign of hormonal disorder. To distinguish those women with definable hormonal disorders from women with medically insignificant hypertrichosis is the responsibility of the physician. The purpose of this chapter is not to discuss all the various interesting and important research that has been performed in this field but to present a clinical approach to the evaluation of the hirsute female.

DEFINITION

In order to separate potentially hormonally abnormal hirsute women from those with medically insignificant increases in hair, I accept the definition of hirsutism as the profuse growth of terminal hair on the chin and/or mustache area in women, usually in the 15- to 40-year age group. Terminal hair is thick hair, as contrasted with vellus hair, which is fine hair. It should be noted that this definition excludes an increase in sideburn hair from the category of medically significant hirsutism. It is the author's experience that increased sideburn hair is frequently found in women with a Mediterranean Basin background and is genetic in etiology. Thus in women with only increased sideburn hair, hormonal studies are of limited value. There is not universal acceptance of this proposed definition of hirsutism.

OUTPATIENT EVALUATION

When a patient presents in the physician's office with the complaint of hirsutism, a careful history and a physical examination (including a pelvic examination) must be performed. There are several points that must be noted in the history, such as the onset of the hair growth, location of the hair, depilatory methods used, natural history of the hair (whether it is getting worse), and its relation to menarche. Most individuals with the usual types of hirsutism will note that the onset was perimenarchal, often starting on the chin and mustache area and later spreading laterally from the chin, eventually involving the skin over the sternum and up the linea alba.

A careful drug history must be taken not only to rule out medications as a cause of the hirsutism but also because many compounds will interfere with the endocrine evaluation (vide infra). Common causes of hirsutism are such drugs as diphenylhydantoin and phenothiazines, but the list of medications causing hirsutism is almost endless, and thus any medication that the patient has been ingesting should be looked up in the literature to rule it out as a cause of hirsutism.

Many women with hirsutism have menstrual irregularities, and thus a detailed menstrual history must be obtained. Medically significant hirsutism may be present even if the menses are completely normal. A perfectly normal menstrual history strongly argues against ovarian disorders as being etiologic in causing the hirsutism.

Acne vulgaris is an androgen-dependent disorder and is frequently found accompanying hirsutism. In some cases the acne may have responded favorably to estrogen or glucocorticoid administration. This information is important, for it may later help to determine the appropriate therapy for the hirsutism.

Thyroid dysfunction may cause hirsutism, and therefore the patient should be carefully questioned as to hyperthyroid and hypothyroid symptoms. Replacement doses of thyroid hormones do not cause hirsutism.

A careful historical search should be performed to uncover any history of hirsutism in the patient's mother, aunts, or sisters. If possible, their menstrual histories should be ascertained, as well as their pregnancy histories. There is little question that hirsutism is prominent in certain families, although authorities differ on the reasons for this.

A complete physical examination should be performed on the patient, with particular emphasis on the integument. The patient may complain of hypertrichosis, but it is the role of the physician to make the diagnosis of medically significant hirsutism. Many women will present in the physician's office complaining of profuse hair growth, and yet physical diagnosis will fail to confirm the presence of significant hirsutism. Some of these patients are having social problems that they attempt to attribute to their hirsutism, when in reality there is no hirsutism. Thus if significant hirsutism is not found on physical examination, endocrine evaluation will prove fruitless and may actually be harmful, for it could reinforce the patient's false belief that she has hirsutism and thus allow her to avoid dealing with the actual psychosocial problem.

In many women, one look at the face confirms the diagnosis of hirsutism. There are other women who complain of hirsutism and who have some terminal hair on the chin or mustache area, but there is the question of how profuse the hirsutism is. Doubt may exist in the mind of the physician as to whether the hirsutism is severe enough to merit an extensive endocrinologic evaluation. Some important clues that enable one to answer this question are the presence or absence of hair over the sternum and/or linea alba and the menstrual history. Equivocal facial hair associated with menstrual irregularities should be endocrinologically evaluated. Profuse terminal hair over the sternum and/or linea alba in the presence of equivocal facial hair should be endocrinologically evaluated. Hair around the areolae has, in my experience, not proved to be significant. Severe nodulocystic acne should also influence one toward an endocrinologic evaluation.

On the physical examination it is important to differentiate hirsutism from virilism. Hirsutism, as defined above, may be found either alone or in association with virilism.

Evaluation and Therapy of the Hirsute Female

Virilism usually implies a high level of a strong androgen for a long time. In virilism, besides hirsutism, one often finds male-pattern scalp balding, clitoromegaly, and development of male-pattern masculature. The virilism workup differs somewhat from the hirsutism workup and will not be discussed in this chapter.

The pelvic examination is necessary not only to rule out the occasional male pseudohermaphrodite who might present with the complaint of hirsutism but also to determine ovarian size. Some of the patients are obese, and thus the pelvic examination might not be ideal to assess ovarian size. Contrary to popular belief, most women with hirsutism are not obese; in my experience only one-third have been significantly overweight.

OUTPATIENT LABORATORY STUDIES

When the physician is convinced by the history and physical examination that the patient has hirsutism, he then orders certain hormonal studies. These studies vary to some extent with the personal bias of the individual practitioner, but as a minimum I make the following tests: (1) serum luteinizing hormone (LH) and testosterone determinations and (2) standard 2-mg dexamethasone suppression test; if examination leads one to suspect some other disorder, such as thyroid dysfunction, then the necessary tests are also obtained.

Serum LH

The serum LH value is now easily available from commercial laboratories throughout the United States. It is performed by radioimmunoassay and is highly accurate. An elevated serum LH level in conjunction with a pelvic examination disclosing enlarged ovaries is virtually diagnostic of Stein-Leventhal syndrome. Patients who do not have elevated serum LH values may also have Stein-Leventhal syndrome, and in these instances it can be definitively diagnosed only by an abdominal surgical procedure such as laparoscopy or culdoscopy.

Serum Testosterone

Serum and plasma testosterone levels are available throughout the country. The hormone is measured by radioimmunoassay. Most patients with hirsutism have normal or slightly elevated testosterone levels. Higher testosterone values are found in Stein-Leventhal syndrome. Very high testosterone determinations indicate that one should strongly consider the possibility of an ovarian or adrenocortical neoplasm.

Standard 2-Mg Dexamethasone Suppression Test

The methodology for performing this test is described in detail in Appendix A. The purpose of this test is to rule out Cushing's syndrome, which may be caused by bilateral adrenocortical hyperplasia, adrenocortical adenoma, or adrenocortical carcinoma. If Cushing's syndrome is present, 24-hr urinary excretion of 17-hydroxycorticosteroids will not suppress to 4 mg or less on the dexamethasone test. It is also possible that an adrenocortical neoplasm secreting predominantly androgens and not glucocorticoids is present. Patients with this type of lesion will usually exhibit markedly elevated 17-ketosteroids, which are resistant to dexamethasone suppression. If the dexamethasone suppression test is abnormal, the patient should be admitted to the hospital for evaluation for Cushing's syndrome (see Chapter 5).

INPATIENT STUDIES

If the outpatient studies previously discussed are not diagnostic and the 2-mg dexamethasone suppression test is within normal limits, I then admit the patient to the hospital for more definitive studies. (If the 2-mg dexamethasone test was abnormal, the patient should be evaluated for Cushing's syndrome.) It is my belief that every attempt must be made to find an etiology for the hirsutism, even though in about 40 percent of women no definite cause can be ascertained. To achieve this goal the patient is subjected to a 24-hr ACTH (given as Cortrosyn) infusion, with measurement of urinary tetrahydro S (THS) and pregnanetriol. If the patient has a history of abnormal menses, a laparoscopy is also performed. The purpose of these tests is to attempt to define and separate adrenocortical abnormalities from ovarian hormonal abnormalities.

Partial Adrenogenital Syndrome

The adrenocortical enzyme deficiencies of 11- or 21-hydroxylation usually present in the pediatric age group, and hirsutism is one of their manifestations. Recently it has become apparent that partial deficiencies of 11- or 21-hydroxylation may appear in the adult female with hirsutism and/or acne as the only clinical findings. It is to diagnose the partial 11- or 21-hydroxylase deficiencies that urinary THS and pregnanetriol are measured. Urinary THS elevation implies an 11-hydroxylase deficiency, whereas pregnanetriol elevation implies a 21-hydroxylase deficiency. Basal 24-hr urinary measurements of THS and pregnanetriol in adult hirsute females show little difference from the results obtained in normal nonhirsute females. It is only by constantly stressing the adrenal cortex for 24 hr with ACTH (given as Cortrosyn) that the significant differences from normal women can be detected.

ACTH 24-hr Infusion

The patient is admitted to the hospital for performance of a 24-hr ACTH infusion (see Appendix B for details of performance of test), and a 24-hr urine is collected simultaneously with the infusion. The urine is assayed for creatinine, 17-ketosteroids, 17-hydroxycorticosteroids, THS, and pregnanetriol. The results obtained are compared to those determined in normal nonhirsute women.[1] Normal women excrete less than 3.3 mg of pregnanetriol and less than 4.6 mg of THS in response to the 24-hr ACTH infusion. Hirsute women with excretions of either THS or pregnanetriol greater than two standard deviations from the mean of those exhibited by control women are classified as probably having a partial adrenogenital syndrome.

Laparoscopy

Laparoscopy should be performed on all hirsute women with menstrual irregularities in whom physical diagnosis and laboratory studies have not made a definite diagnosis of Stein-Leventhal syndrome. It is possible that the classic features of Stein-Leventhal syndrome may be absent and the individual still have enlarged polycystic ovaries. Thus it is the author's opinion that laparoscopy is indicated in women with hirsutism and menstrual irregularities. I do not have laparoscopy performed in women with hirsutism and normal menses.

THERAPY

Stein-Leventhal Syndrome

If the diagnosis of Stein-Leventhal syndrome has been made and fertility is not currently desired, many gynecologists give the patient a trial of cyclical estrogen therapy. If hirsutism is the only abnormality being treated, it is frequently necessary to treat for a year before a decision can be reached as to therapeutic effect. Unfortunately, there is no good way yet available to quantitate hair growth, and thus one is forced to rely on clinical impression. If fertility is desired, then a trial of clomiphene is indicated.

Partial Adrenogenital Syndrome

If the diagnosis of either an 11- or 21-hydroxylase deficiency has been made, then the patient is placed on prednisone 5 mg orally twice a day. The patient should be kept on this dosage for a year before a decision can be made as to its effect on the hirsutism. If the patient has menstrual irregularities or acne, improvement in these parameters may portend a good response with the hirsutism. It is my experience in women of this age group that side effects with this dosage of prednisone are few. The prednisone can be withdrawn at the end of the therapy period by gradual tapering over a 3-week period. If the hirsutism has responded to the prednisone, but on discontinuing the prednisone it recurs, it may be necessary to reinstitute prednisone.

Idiopathic Hirsutism

If no diagnosis as to the etiology of the hirsutism can be determined, the woman is classified as having idiopathic hirsutism. The diagnosis should be discussed with the patient, and it should be the patient's decision whether hormonal therapy is tried empirically.

Electrolysis

All patients with hirsutism, whether hormonally related or not, should have electrolysis performed on the superfluous hair. The electrology treatments should be used in conjunction with hormonal therapy. Electrolysis is directed against hair that is already present and growing, whereas hormonal therapy attempts to suppress growth of new hair.

SUMMARY

Hirsutism is a widespread problem in the United States, and in 40 percent of these patients the routinely available tests cannot determine an etiology. These patients should undergo complete endocrinologic evaluation and this chapter has attempted to present one program for such clinical evaluation of the hirsute female. Therapy should be initiated only after the hormonal evaluation has been completed.

REFERENCES

1. Rose LI, Newmark SR, Strauss JD et al: Adrenocortical hydroxylase deficiencies in acne vulgaris. Invest Dermatol 66:342–326, 1976
2. Taymore ML, Berger MJ: Polycystic ovary syndrome (Stein-Leventhal syndrome), in Gold JJ (ed): Gynecologic Endocrinology (ed 2). New York, Harper & Row, 1975, pp 461–477
3. Segre EJ: Androgens, Virilization and the Hirsute Female. Springfield, Ill, Charles C Thomas, 1967
4. Kischner MA: Androgen production and hirsutism, in Kryston LJ, Shaw RA (eds): Endocrinology and Diabetes. New York, Grune & Stratton, 1975, pp 299–310
5. Newmark S, Dluhy RG, Williams GH et al: Partial 11- and 21-hydroxylase deficiencies in hirsute females. Am J Obstet Gynecol (in press)

Evaluation and Therapy of the Hirsute Female

APPENDIX A

Dexamethasone Suppression Test — 2 mg

Purpose:

A definitive test to rule out Cushing's syndrome.

Preparation:
1. Patient must not be on any drugs or medications for at least 2 days prior to the test and during performance of the test.
2. No stressful procedures should be performed on the patient while the test is in progress.

Equipment:
1. Dexamethasone 0.5 mg p.o. × 8 doses.
2. Three 24-hr urine containers with 25 ml glacial acetic acid in each container as preservative.

Procedure:

Day 1: Starting at 8 A.M. collect 24-hr urine 17-ketosteroids (17-KS), 17-hydroxycorticosteroids (17-OHCS), creatinine, urinary free F (cortisol), and total volume for baseline values.

Day 2: Starting at 8 A.M. give dexamethasone 0.5 mg p.o. every 6 hr. Collect 24-hr urine as on day 1.

Day 3: Continue dexamethasone 0.5 mg p.o. every 6 hr. Collect 24-hr urine as on day 1.

Interpretation:
1. Normal individuals will have 17-OHCS of 1.5–13 mg/24 hr on day 1.
2. Normal individuals will have 17-KS of 3–15 mg/24 hr in males and 2–10 mg/24 hr in females.
3. Normal individuals will suppress urinary 17-OHCS excretion to 3.5 mg/24 hr or less on either day 2 or day 3 of the test. If this occurs, Cushing's syndrome has been ruled out.
4. Individuals with Cushing's syndrome will have urinary free F on day 1 greater than 90 μg/24 hr.
5. If urinary 17-OHCS excretion is greater than 4.0 mg/24 hr on day 3, the patient probably has Cushing's syndrome, and further investigative tests are indicated, i.e., the 8-mg dexamethasone test.

APPENDIX B

Cortrosyn Infusion (Time 24–48 hr)

Purpose:
To investigate the response of the adrenal cortex to a continuous 24-hr ACTH stimulation. (Cortrosyn is the synthetic $\alpha^{1\text{-}24}$-ACTH).

Indications:
Test is performed in patients with hirsutism and/or acne.

Equipment:

1. Cortrosyn 25 units, 2 vials (4 vials for 48 hr).
2. IV solution 500 cc, 2 bottles (4 bottles for 48 hr).
3. Solution administration set with minidrip.
4. #19 scalp vein needle, or
5. #20 angio cath.
6. Alcohol sponges
7. Tape, 1 in.
8. Receptacle for 24-hr urine with preservative.

Medication:

1. Dosage: 2 vials of Cortrosyn per 24 hr, usually administered as 25 units/500 cc IV starting at 12 hr.
2. IV solution: saline 0.9 percent, D_5W (in cases where N.S. is contraindicated).

Procedure:
The dose is administered evenly over a 24-hr period intravenously. This is done by infusing 25 units of Cortrosyn in 500 cc IV solution over consecutive 12-hr periods.

Concomitant with the Cortrosyn infusions, 24-hr urines are collected for total volume, creatinine, 17-ketosteroids, 17-hydroxycorticosteroids, tetrahydro S (THS), and pregnanetriol

Interpretation:
To rule out adrenocortical insufficiency:

	First Day (mg 17-OHCS/24 hr)
Normals	18 or >
Primary adrenocortical insufficiency	0–4
Secondary adrenocortical insufficiency	5–12

To rule out partial 21- or 11-hydroxylase enzyme deficiencies:

	THS	Pregnanetriol
Normals	0–4.7	0–3.3
21-Hydroxylase blocks	0–4.7	> 3.3
11-Hydroxylase blocks	> 4.7	0–3.3

Note: Patients with 11-hydroxylase deficiencies may also elevate their pregnanetriol excretions on ACTH and therefore both THS and pregnanetriol may be elevated.

Caution: (1) Not to be used in patients suspected of having Cushing's disease. (2) The patient is given dexamethasone 0.5 mg b.i.d. to prevent any crisis from occurring in patients suspected of having Addison's disease.

Charles Y.C. Pak, Donald Barilla,
Henry Bone, and Cheryl Northcutt

9
Medical Management of Renal Calculi

Recurrent nephrolithiasis is a common medical disorder that affects nearly 0.3 percent of the population in the United States. Recently, significant strides have been made toward the resolution of two question: Why do stones form in vitro? Why are certain patients more prone to develop stones? Specifically, we need to know the physicochemical factors concerned with stone formation and whether there are underlying metabolic defects that predispose to nephrolithiasis. Examination of these questions of why stones form in vitro and in vivo has led to the development of a rational mode of therapy. We shall review these recent trends for the most commonly occurring stones — those that contain calcium.

PHYSICAL CHEMISTRY OF STONE FORMATION

Renal stones probably begin from the crystal nidus, formed either by spontaneous precipitation[1] or in an organic matrix.[2] Once formed, the nidus may grow into a macroscopic stone of homogeneous composition by processes of crystal growth[3] and crystal aggregation[4] or a stone of heterogeneous composition by epitaxial growth.[5] Several epitaxial growth relationships are now recognized. Thus, brushite ($CaHPO_4 \cdot 2H_2O$), hydroxyapatite, and monosodium urate monohydrate may serve as seeds for the crystallization of Ca oxalate.[5-7] Techniques have now been developed to quantitate these processes. For example, the activity product ratio (APR) expresses the state of saturation, where the value 1 indicates saturation, values greater than 1 indicate supersaturation, and values less than 1 indicate undersaturation.[8] The crystal nidus may form when the APR exceeds the formation product ratio (FPR).

An essential requirement for the formation of stones is persistent passage of urine supersaturated with respect to the constituents of stones, since nucleation and subsequent growth of nidus cannot proceed in undersaturated urine. Thus urine specimens from patients with Ca urolithiasis have usually been found to be supersaturated with respect to both brushite and Ca oxalate, whereas those from control subjects are often undersaturated.[8,9]

Supported by USPHS grants R01-AM-16016, M01-RR-00633, and P01-HL-11662.

A major determinant for supersaturation with respect to Ca phosphate and Ca oxalate is a high urinary concentration of Ca. Thus the urinary APRs of brushite and Ca oxalate are directly dependent on the urinary concentration of CA.[8,9]

CAUSES OF HYPERCALCIURIA

Hypercalciuria is frequently encountered among patients with Ca urolithiasis.[10] It may be etiologically important in stone formation, because it is known to have an association with the supersaturated state with respect to brushite and oxalate. For this reason our initial effort has been directed at delineating the causes of hypercalciuria.

Three major causes of hypercalciuria, each associated with nephrolithiasis, have been recognized.[10] In resorptive hypercalciuria, characterized by primary hyperparathyroidism, there is excessive resorption of bone because of hypersecretion of parathyroid hormone (PTH) by abnormal parathyroid tissue (usually adenomatous gland). There may be intestinal hyperabsorption of Ca, probably consequent to PTH-dependent stimulation of synthesis of $1\alpha,25$-dihydroxycholecalciferol [$1\alpha,25$-$(OH)_2D$].[11] These combined effects increase the circulating concentration of Ca and the renal filtered load of Ca. The occurrence of hypercalciuria seems paradoxic, since the primary renal action of PTH is stimulation of renal tubular reabsorption of Ca. However, hypercalciuria is often encountered in primary hyperparathyroidism because the increase in the renal filtered load of Ca is usually predominant.

In absorptive hypercalciuria there is primary intestinal hyperabsorption of Ca. The consequent increase in the circulating concentration of Ca augments the renal filtered load of Ca and suppresses parathyroid function. Hypercalciuria ensues because of the increased renal filtered load of Ca and reduced renal tubular reabsorption of Ca consequent to parathyroid suppression.

The excessive renal loss of Ca compensates for the high Ca absorption from the intestinal tract and maintains serum concentration of Ca in the normal range. The cause for intestinal hyperabsorption of Ca is not known. Our preliminary studies indicate that the plasma concentration of $1\alpha,25$-$(OH)_2D$ is elevated in approximately one-third of patients with absorptive hypercalciuria and normal in the remaining two-thirds. However, increased synthesis of $1\alpha,25$-$(OH)_2D$ is not likely the cause for high intestinal absorption of Ca. When patients with absorptive hypercalciuria are given diphenylhydantoin, intestinal absorption of Ca is not significantly altered, even though the circulating concentration of $1\alpha,25$-$(OH)_2D$ is reduced. Further, hypersensitivity to vitamin D probably cannot account for the high intestinal absorption of Ca in this condition, since prednisone does not lower intestinal Ca absorption.

In renal hypercalciuria[10,12] the primary abnormality is impairment in renal tubular reabsorption of Ca. The consequent reduction in the circulating concentration of Ca stimulates parathyroid function. There may be excessive mobilization of Ca from bone and enhanced intestinal absorption of Ca from the PTH excess. These effects restore serum Ca to the normal range. Unlike the situation in primary hyperparathyroidism, serum Ca is normal, and the state of hyperparathyroidism is secondary.

The syndromes of absorptive hypercalciuria and renal hypercalciuria are probably the major variants of idiopathic hypercalciuria. Absorptive hypercalciuria shares with idiopathic hypercalciuria the following features: a preponderance of male subjects over female

Table 9-1
Clinical Data

	No. Patients	Percentage with Stones
Primary hyperparathyroidism	74	
with stones	21	17.9
Absorptive hypercalciuria (type I)	40	34.2
Absorptive hypercalciuria (type II)	19	16.2
Renal hypercalciuria	16	13.7
Normocalciuric nephrolithiasis	21	17.9

subjects and recurrent Ca urolithiasis as the only recognizable clinical manifestation. In renal hypercalciuria the two sexes are equally affected, and bone disease as well as Ca urolithiasis may be present.

DIAGNOSTIC CRITERIA FOR HYPERCALCIURIAS

A reliable method for the differentiation of the three forms of hypercalciuria has been developed.[10,13] While patients were maintained on a constant liquid synthetic diet containing 400 mg Ca, 800 mg P, and 100 mEq Na per day, accurate measures of parathyroid function and Ca metabolism were obtained. From July 1, 1972, to October 1, 1975, 117 patients with recurrent Ca urolithiasis were evaluated (Table 9-1). Primary hyperparathyroidism accounted for 13 percent, absorptive hypercalciuria 50 percent, and renal hypercalciuria 14 percent.

Absorptive hypercalciuria consisted of two forms[6,13]: In absorptive hypercalciuria type I there was excessive renal excretion of Ca at all levels of Ca intake. In absorptive hypercalciuria type II, enhanced Ca excretion was demonstrated only at a high intake of Ca. Eighteen percent of patients were found to have no demonstrable abnormality of Ca metabolism (normocalciuric nephrolithiasis). However, many of them had hyperuricosuria. They probably suffered from the disorder described by Coe and Raisen[14] in which patients with normocalciuria and hyperuricosuria form Ca stones. The majority of patients with primary hyperparathyroidism and stones had excessive renal excretion of Ca. Hypercalciuria was found in nearly 80 percent of all patients with Ca urolithiasis.

In primary hyperparathyroidism (PHPT) serum Ca concentration was elevated in the majority of cases (Fig. 9-1). Even though serum Ca was normal in 16 percent of cases, hypercalciuria was found prior to this evaluation in all cases. Serum concentration of P was low in only 18 percent of cases; it was within the normal range in the majority of cases. Hypercalciuria (urinary Ca greater than 200 mg/day) was encountered in 64 percent of cases. Urinary Ca exceeded the intake of 400 mg/day in 12 percent of cases. In absorptive hypercalciuria (AH), renal hypercalciuria (RH), and normocalciuric nephrolithiasis (NN) serum concentrations of Ca and P were within the normal range. In AH type I, urinary Ca was greater than 200 mg/day, but less than the intake of 400 mg/day. In AH type II and in NN, urinary Ca was within the normal range. In RH, urinary Ca was high or high normal.

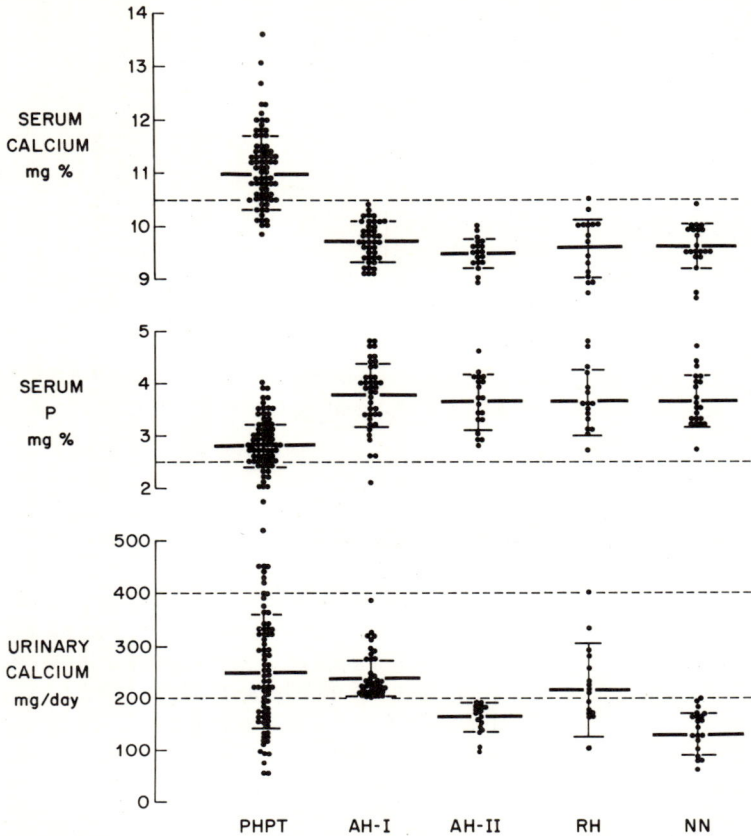

Fig. 9–1. Serum Ca, serum P, and urinary Ca in primary hyperparathyroidism (PHPT), absorptive hypercalciuria type I (AH-I), absorptive hypercalciuria type II (AH-II), renal hypercalciuria (RH), and normocalciuric nephrolithiasis (NN). The dashed horizontal lines indicate upper range for serum Ca and lower range for serum P. For urinary Ca, the dashed lines represent the intake of 400 mg/day and the upper range of normal of 200 mg/day. Bars represent means ± SD.

In PHPT and in secondary hyperparathyroidism of RH, intestinal Ca absorption (fractional Ca absorption) from an oral load of 100 mg was elevated in approximately 70 percent of cases (Fig. 9–2). Whereas it was invariably high in AH type I, it was increased in only some of the patients with AH type II and NN. In PHPT and RH, urinary Ca (Ca_{UV}) exceeded absorbed Ca (Ca_A) in approximately 40 percent and 25 percent of cases, respectively, a fact reflecting a state of negative Ca balance.[10] In other groups, absorbed Ca usually exceeded urinary Ca.

During the fasting state, urinary Ca may reflect the extent of mobilization of Ca from bone, since there is no significant absorption of Ca from the intestinal tract.[15] Fasting urinary Ca was invariably high in RH and was elevated in 68 percent of cases of PHPT (Fig. 9–3). It was usually normal in other groups. Bone density in the distal third of the radius by ^{125}I-photon absorption[16] was low (as compared to values in age- and sex-matched control subjects) in 30 percent of cases of PHPT and in 19 percent of cases of RH. The results suggest that there may be excessive resorption of bone, probably from PTH excess in these two conditions.

Medical Management of Renal Calculi

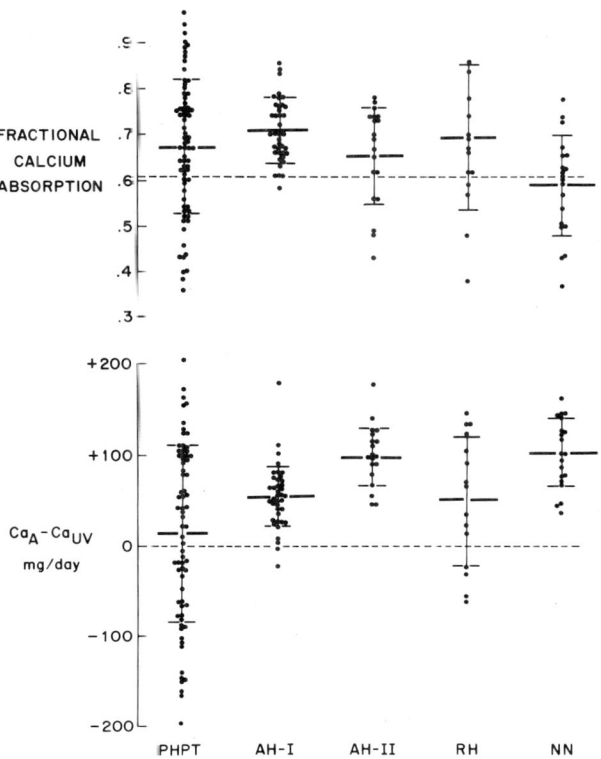

Fig. 9-2. Fractional Ca absorption and $Ca_A - Ca_{UV}$. The upper range of normal for fractional Ca absorption is given by the dashed horizontal line. $Ca_A - Ca_{UV}$ represents the difference between absorbed and excreted Ca. Bars represent means ± SD.

Urinary cyclic AMP (cAMP) was measured in 24-hr samples obtained under constant dietary regimen.[10] It was elevated in 67 percent of cases of PHPT and in 44 percent of cases of RH (Fig. 9-4). It was normal or low in other groups. The results are consistent with the previous demonstration that serum immunoreactive PTH is often elevated in PHPT[10] and RH[12] and normal or low in AH and NN.[10]

The majority of patients also underwent studies of fasting and Ca load.[13] A 2-hr fasting urine sample following an overnight fast and a 4-hr urine sample following an oral load of 1 g Ca were obtained; the samples were assayed for Ca, creatinine, and cAMP. This test was essential in the diagnosis of AH type II and was helpful in the diagnosis of renal hypercalciuria. In patients with AH type II and patients with NN the 24-hr urinary Ca was within the normal range (Fig. 9-1). However, following oral load of an excess of Ca there was an exaggerated increase in urinary Ca in patients with AH type II (Fig. 9-5), a fact suggesting that these patients hyperabsorb Ca from the intestinal tract. In patients with NN the response to Ca load was normal. Urinary cAMP did not change significantly following Ca load (as compared to fasting values) in PHPT (Fig. 9-6). In patients with RH, urinary cAMP, which was high in 6 of 11 patients during fast, returned toward normal following oral Ca load, a finding indicating suppressibility of PTH secretion.[13] The typical features of the three forms of hypercalciuria and NN are presented in Table 9-2.

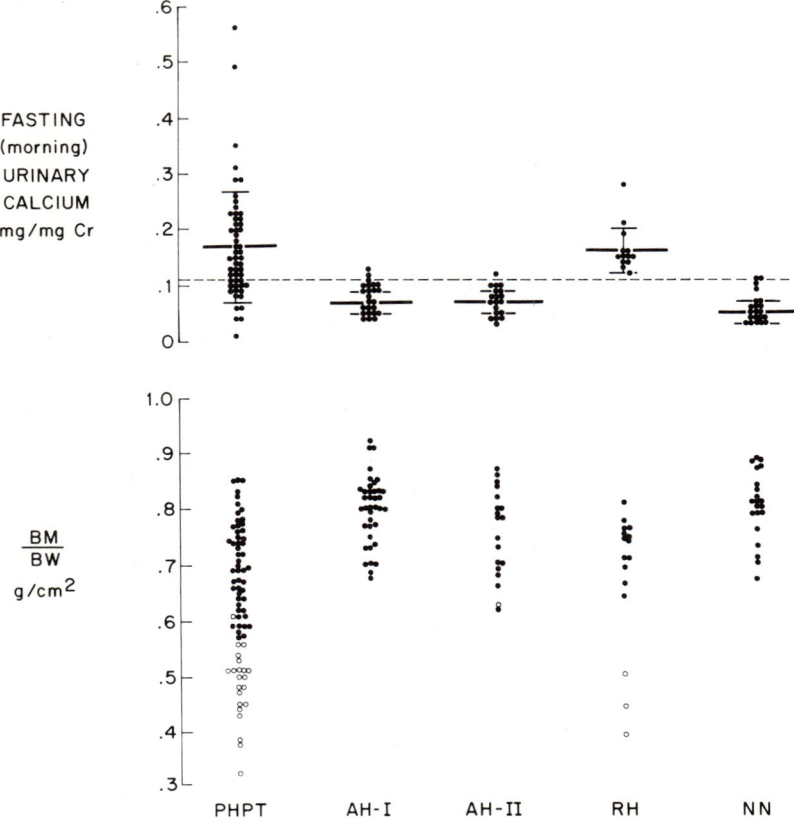

Fig. 9-3. Fasting urinary Ca and bone density (BM/BW). The dashed horizontal line indicates the upper range of normal for fasting urinary Ca following an overnight fast. Open circles for density represent values that are below 4th percentile of age- and sex-matched values for control subjects. Bars represent means ± SD.

THERAPEUTIC CONSIDERATIONS

Recent advances in the physical chemistry of renal stone formation[9] have led to a better understanding of the mechanisms by which certain drugs recommended for renal stones exert their action in vitro.[6] An elucidation of the causes of hypercalciuria[10,12] has facilitated the development of a rational basis for therapy based on correcting the underlying disorder. The following discussion gives a review of our current understanding of the mechanisms of action in vitro and in vivo and a listing of the clinical indications for various drugs that are currently available for control of Ca urolithiasis. This discussion includes two drugs that are investigational in the United States: sodium cellulose phosphate and diphosphonate.

Sodium Cellulose Phosphate

Sodium cellulose phosphate[17] is a nonabsorbable ion-exchange resin with high affinity for Ca^{++}. When it is given orally with meals, part of the dietary Ca may become bound to the resin by exchanging for Na. It therefore effectively inhibits the intestinal

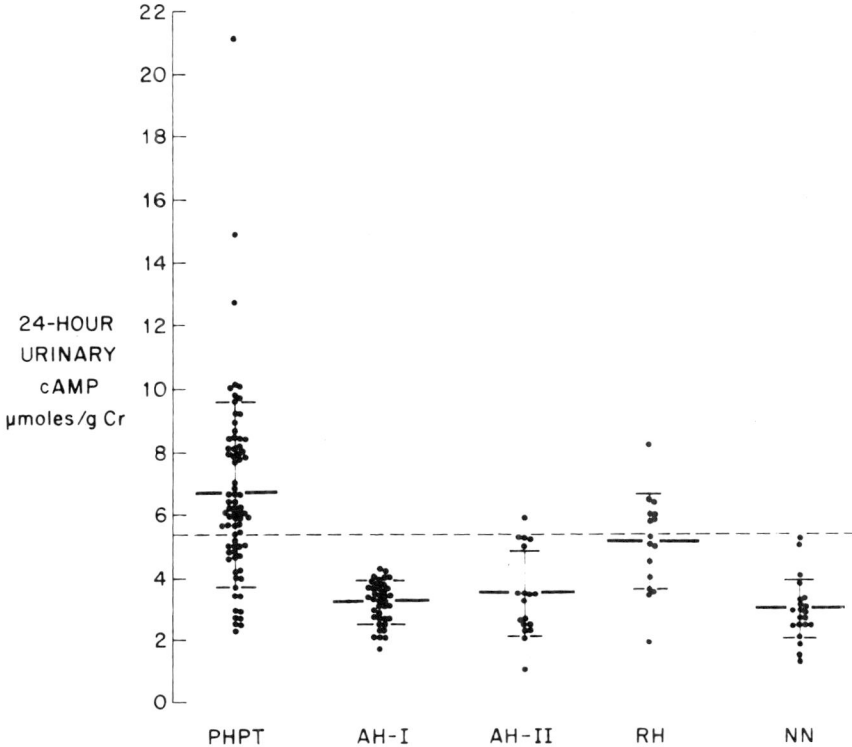

Fig. 9-4. Urinary cyclic AMP (24-hr). Cyclic AMP is expressed relative to urinary creatinine (Cr). The dashed horizontal line indicates upper range of normal. Bars represent means ± SD.

absorption of Ca. It is currently the drug of choice for hypercalciuria, since it may effectively correct both intestinal hyperabsorption of Ca and hypercalciuria.[10,17]

The effects of this therapy on the renal excretion of electrolytes and on the propensity for crystallization of calcium phosphate and calcium oxalate are well known. In patients with absorptive hypercalciuria who are maintained on a low-Ca diet (approximately 400 mg Ca per day), sodium cellulose phosphate (1.5 g P per day) decreases urinary Ca by 100–200 mg/day and increases urinary P by 200–400 mg/day.[10,17] Since the decrease in urinary Ca is predominant, the urinary activity product ratio (state of saturation) of brushite decreases, often from supersaturation to undersaturation.[17]

During treatment, urinary oxalate increases, probably from the binding of Ca in the intestinal tract, which leaves more oxalate available for absorption.[18] However, because the fall in urinary Ca is usually greater, the urinary APR (state of saturation) decreases or does not change significantly.

The treatment does not significantly alter renal excretion of pyrophosphate, sulfate, or citrate.[17] The urinary FPRs (limits of metastability) and crystal growth of brushite and Ca oxalate are not significantly changed.[18]

Orthophosphates

Unlike sodium cellulose phosphate, which is not absorbable, the sodium and potassium salts of orthophosphate are absorbable by virtue of their high solubility. When given orally, orthophosphates markedly increase urinary P and cause a moderate decrease in

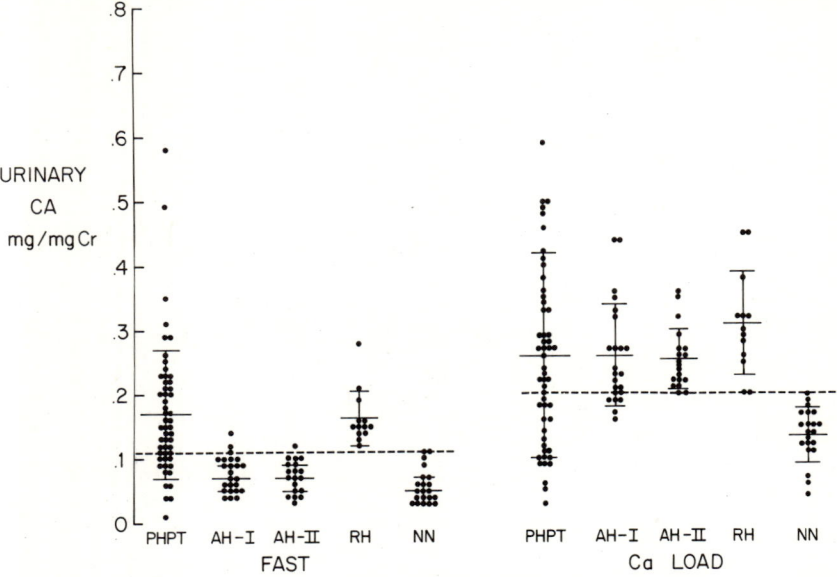

Fig. 9-5. Urinary Ca during fast and following oral load of 1 g Ca. Urinary Ca is expressed relative to urinary Cr. Dashed horizontal lines indicate upper range of normal. Bars represent means ± SD.

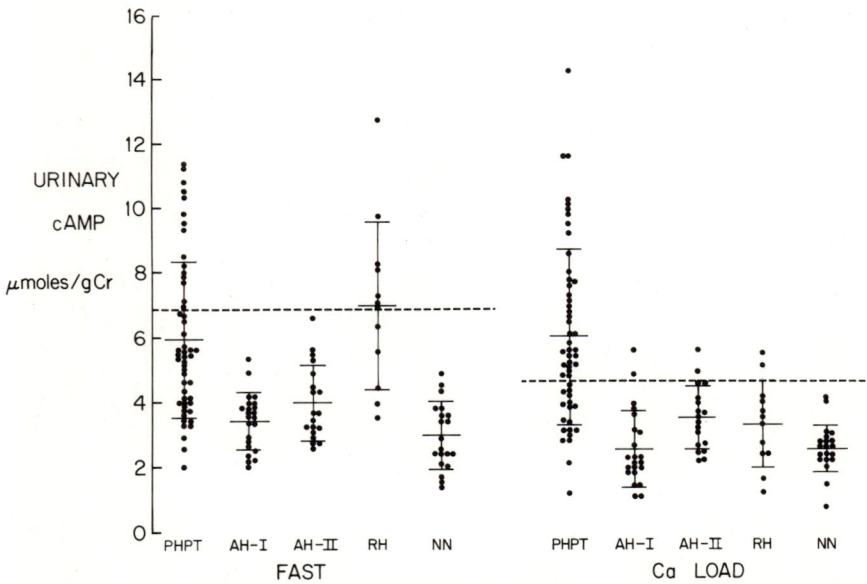

Fig. 9-6. Urinary cyclic AMP during fast and following Ca load. Dashed horizontal lines indicate upper range of values for control subjects. Bars represent means ± SD.

Table 9-2
Diagnostic Criteria for Hypercalciurias and Normocalciuric Nephrolithiasis

	PHPT	AH-I	AH-II	RH	NN
Serum Ca	▲*	N	N	N	N
Serum P	N/▼	N	N	N	N
Urinary Ca (24-hr)	N/▲	▲	N	N/▲	N
Urinary Ca after Ca load	▲	▲	▲	N/▲	N
Urinary Ca during fast	▲	N	N	▲	N
Urinary cAMP (24-hr)	▲	N	N	▲	N
Urinary cAMP after Ca load	▲	N	N	N	N

*Notations: ▲ increase; ▼ decrease; N normal; N/▲ normal or increase; N/▼ normal or decrease.

urinary Ca.[19] The exact mechanism for the latter effect is not known. Because the increase in urinary P is predominant, the urinary APR of brushite increases.[19] Furthermore, orthophosphates promote renal excretion of inhibitors of crystallization, including pyrophosphate.[20] Thus, despite increased saturation with respect to brushite, the treatment may be effective because it may retard nucleation and crystal growth of brushite and Ca oxalate.[19]

Potential hazards of this therapy[21,22] include soft-tissue calcification, renal functional deterioration, and parathyroid stimulation. These potential side effects should be carefully considered before subjecting patients to long-term treatment. Orthophosphates might be indicated in certain patients with absorptive hypercalciuria in whom intestinal hyperabsorption of Ca may have resulted from primary impairment in renal tubular reabsorption of P (renal leak) and overproduction of $1\alpha,25\text{-}(OH)_2D$.[23]

Thiazides

Thiazides are unique among diuretics in their ability to reduce renal excretion of Ca.[12] In renal hypercalciuria, thiazides are particularly useful, since they may restore renal leak of Ca, secondary hyperparathyroidism, and intestinal hyperabsorption of Ca.

During treatment, urinary APRs (states of saturation) of brushite and Ca oxalate usually decrease, probably because of the fall in urinary Ca. Thiazides also promote renal excretion of pyrophosphate and zinc.[24] Thus nucleation and crystal growth of brushite and Ca oxalate are usually retarded.

Diphosphonates

Diphosphonates, synthetic analogues of pyrophosphate, are resistant to degradation by pyrophosphatase. When added to real or "artificial" urine in vitro, diphosphonates have been shown to inhibit nucleation and crystal growth of brushite[25] and Ca oxalate,[3] crystal aggregation of Ca oxalate, and heterogeneous nucleation of Ca oxalate by monosodium urate or hydroxyapatite.[6] When disodium ethane-1-hydroxy-1,1-diphosphonate (EHDP) is given orally to patients with Ca urolithiasis,[26] similar inhibitions of nucleation and crystal growth of brushite and Ca oxalate in urine are often produced.

In the urine of some stone-forming patients, low FPRs and high rates of crystal growth of brushite and Ca oxalate are found;[9] these facts suggest defective renal excretion of inhibitors of crystallization or excretion in large amounts of "promoters" of crystallization. Treatment of these patients with disphosphonates might be indicated, as it will probably reverse the above abnormalities. Unfortunately, this therapy potentially may be complicated by serious side effects, including osteomalacia.[27]

REFERENCES

1. Pak CYC, Eanes ED, Ruskin B: Spontaneous precipitation of brushite: Evidence that brushite is the nidus of renal stones originating as calcium phosphate. Proc Natl Acad Sci USA 68:1456, 1971
2. Pak CYC, Ruskin B: Calcification of collagen by urine in vitro: Dependence on the degree of saturation of urine with respect to brushite. J Clin Invest 49:2353, 1970
3. Pak CYC, Ohata M, Holt K: Effect of diphosphonate on crystallization of calcium oxalate in vitro. Kidney Int 7:154, 1975
4. Robertson WG: A method for measuring calcium crystalluria. Clin Chim Acta 20:105, 1969
5. Pak CYC, Arnold LH: Heterogeneous nucleation of calcium oxalate by seeds of monosodium urate. Proc Soc Exp Biol Med 149:930, 1975
6. Pak CYC: Physicochemical and clinical aspects of nephrolithiasis, in Finlayson B, Thomas W (eds): Symp Intern Colloq Renal Lithiasis. Gainesville, University of Florida, 1975
7. Pak CYC: Quantitative assessment of various forms of therapy for nephrolithiasis. Urinary calculi, in Cifuentes Delatte L, Rapado A, Hodgkinson A (eds): International Symposium on Renal Stone Research. Basel, Karger, 1973, p 177
8. Pak CYC: Physicochemical basis for formation of renal stones of calcium phosphate origin: Calculation of the degree of saturation of urine with respect to brushite. J Clin Invest 48:1914, 1969
9. Pak CYC, Holt K: Nucleation and growth of brushite and calcium oxalate in urine of stone-formers. Metabolism (in press)
10. Pak CYC, Ohata M, Lawrence EC, et al: The hypercalciurias; causes, parathyroid functions and diagnostic criteria. J Clin Invest 54:387, 1974
11. Haussler MR, Bursac KM, Bone H, et al: Increased circulating $1\alpha,25$-dihydroxy-vitamin D_3 in patients with primary hyperparathyroidism. Clin Res 23:322A, 1975
12. Coe FL, Canterbury JM, Firpo JJ, et al: Evidence for secondary hyperparathyroidism in idiopathic hypercalciuria. J Clin Invest 52:134, 1973
13. Pak CYC, Kaplan R, Bone H, et al: A simple test for the diagnosis of absorptive, resorptive and renal hypercalciurias. N Engl J Med 292:497, 1975
14. Coe FL, Raisen L: Allopurinal treatment of uric-acid disorders in calcium stone-formers. Lancet 1:129, 1973
15. Nordin BEC, Peacock M, Wilkinson R: Hypercalciuria and calcium stone disease, in McIntyre I (ed): Clinics in Endocrinology and Metabolism, vol 1, no 1. Philadelphia, WB Saunders, 1972, p 169
16. Cameron JR, Sorenson J: Measurement of bone mineral in vivo—an improved method. Science 142:230, 1963
17. Pak, CYC: Sodium cellulose phosphate: Mechanism of action and effect on mineral metabolism. J Clin Pharmacol 13:15, 1973
18. Hayashi Y, Kaplan RA, Pak CYC: Effect of sodium cellulose phosphate therapy on crystallization of calcium oxalate in urine. Metabolism 24:1273, 1975
19. Pak CYC: Effects of cellulose phosphate and sodium phosphate on formation product and activity product of brushite in urine. Metabolism 21:447, 1972
20. Fleisch H, Bisaz S, Case AD: Effect of orthophosphate on urinary pyrophosphate excretion and the prevention of urolithiasis. Lancet 1:1065, 1964
21. Dudley FJ, Blackburn CRB: Extraskeletal calcification complicating oral neutral-phosphate therapy. Lancet 2:628, 1970
22. Jowsey J, Reiss E, Canterbury JM: Long-term effects of high phosphate intake on parathyroid homone levels and bone metabolism. Acta Orthop Scand 45:801, 1974
23. Shen F, Baylink D, Nelson R, et al: Increased serum 1,25-dihydroxycholecalciferol (1,25-diOHD$_3$) in patients with idiopathic hypercalciuria (IH). Clin Res 23:423A, 1975
24. Pak CYC: Hydrochlorothiazide therapy in nephrolithiasis. Clin Pharmacol Ther 14:209, 1973
25. Ohata M, Pak CYC: The effect of diphosphonate on calcium phosphate crystallization in urine in vitro. Kidney Int 4:401, 1973
26. Ohata M, Pak CYC: Preliminary study of the treatment of nephrolithiasis (calcium stones) with diphosphonate. Metabolism 23:1167, 1974
27. Jowsey J, Riggs BL, Kelly PJ, et al: The treatment of osteoporosis with disodium ethane-1-hydroxy-1,1-diphosphonate. J Lab Clin Med 78:574, 1971

J. Stuart Soeldner
and Byung N. Park

10
Implications from Oral Glucose Tolerance Testing

There is still a good deal of frustration associated with the attempt at early detection of mild diabetes mellitus. Since the introduction early in the twentieth century of the concept of oral glucose administration to detect carbohydrate intolerance, a great number of novel approaches have been suggested to detect carbohydrate intolerance.[1] At this time the oral glucose tolerance test remains the mainstay in the diagnostic armamentarium for detection of mild carbohydrate intolerance states. There have been many innovative approaches to improving early and definitive diagnosis, but it is beyond the scope of this presentation to review all of these. However, it is worthwhile to mention that some of these adaptations of the oral glucose tolerance test have involved a variety of dose administrations, administration of more than one dose of oral glucose in a short period of time, and measurement of materials other than glucose in blood that are altered secondarily to administration of oral glucose.[2-4] In addition, administration of an oral glucose load at various times of the day, other than in the morning after an overnight fast, has been attempted.[5] Although oral glucose administration itself represents a stress, a number of interesting attempts to amplify or magnify this stress by prior administration of adrenal cortical steroids have been made. However, no definitive conclusions have been reached after 20 years of research and clinical studies.[6]

Glucose has also been administered intravenously in an attempt to eliminate some of the variances that are associated with oral administration of any substance.[(7)] The intravenous glucose tolerance test has been extensively evaluated and compared to the oral glucose tolerance test in regard to its capability of detecting early hyperglycemic states, and the consensus is that it is not a better clinical test than the standard oral glucose tolerance test.[8-10]

Finally, other types of carbohydrate and various other pharmacologic materials have been tried, but little clinical diagnostic benefit over the oral glucose tolerance test has been demonstrated.[11] The intravenous tolbutamide test is one such example.[12]

In addition to being the mainstay of diagnosis of early diabetes or hyperglycemic

---

Supported by NIH Grants AM-09748, EY-01421, and AM-05077 and by the Joslin Diabetes Foundation, Inc., Boston, Massachusetts.

states, the oral glucose tolerance test remains a potent tool in the hands of the clinical investigator and the animal researcher. Employing it as a dynamic perturbation on glucose homeostasis, numerous studies have utilized this procedure to gain further insight into the factors that regulate blood sugar levels and the deposition of glucose into various storage forms in various organ systems.

Important metabolic intermediates and factors related to glucose metabolism that have been studied include free fatty acids, lactate, pyruvate, inorganic phosphate levels, insulinlike activity, and serum immunoreactive insulin.

TEST STANDARDIZATION

It is generally accepted that attention to a number of details during the performance of the oral glucose tolerance test is essential for obtaining accurate results. The test is best performed in the morning after the patient has maintained an overnight fast (water allowed) for 10 to 14 hr. A dose of glucose widely employed is 100 g, although in Western Europe 50 g is used frequently. A variety of other dose schedules for administering glucose on the basis of body surface area or on the basis of so much glucose per unit of ideal body weight have been advocated.[2,13] In addition, preparations containing a total glucose or glucose equivalent of approximately 75 g have been utilized, and some studies have shown no significant differences between these preparations and the 100-g glucose dose.[11] This author prefers to utilize the 100-g glucose dose administered in a 10-ounce volume and flavored with a variety of fruit- or cola-flavored metabolically inert materials.

Although the issue of the proper preparation diet for the patient is not completely settled, asking the patient to consume a diet liberal in carbohydrate for 3 days prior to the test is probably most essential. It is quite unclear whether the amount of carbohydrate in the well-balanced diet should amount to 300 g or just exceed 150 g/day.[14,15] Obviously, patients of small body mass require less carbohydrate for adequate preparation than do larger subjects. Weighing the importance of the test against the mild inconvenience of consuming a diet heavy in carbohydrates for such a short period of time, it is probably best to insist on a high-carbohydrate diet preparation until the issue is completely clear.

Table 10–1 illustrates the plan used in the author's laboratory for the key items of patient preparation, as well as a suggested diet to ensure an adequately high carbohydrate intake.

VARIABLES INFLUENCING THE RESULT

Table 10–2 lists most of the identified factors that influence the test results. Those inherited defects and/or factors that lead to diabetes are still essentially unknown. Clearly the prime objective of doing a diagnostic test for detection of early diabetes is to measure the magnitude of impairment of blood sugar homeostasis that is not due to uncontrolled factors such as poor patient preparation, test performance, etc.

The degree of obesity of the patient is a factor that must be considered. It is still not known whether the higher prevalance of abnormal oral glucose tolerance tests in obese individuals represents an amplification by obesity of idiopathic diabetes or whether obesity itself produces mild carbohydrate intolerance that is not really idiopathic diabetes.[16]

A somewhat similar problem exists in regard to age. It has been amply demonstrated

Table 10-1
Preparation for Oral Glucose Tolerance Test: 300-g Carbohydrate Diet

Instructions
1. Follow this diet for 3 full days before test.
2. You will not gain a significant amount of weight after only 3 days on the diet.
3. Any additional food you desire may be eaten (soup, bacon, eggs, meat, vegetables, salads, etc.).
4. If you do not follow this diet as best as you can, it may result in a poor glucose tolerance test.
5. For 12 hours before test, *no food, no liquids other than water, no coffee, no tea,* and *no smoking.*
6. Do not take any medicines (except as directed by us) for 12 hours before test.

Meal Plan
The grams of carbohydrate are in parentheses; you may substitute from lists below.
Breakfast:
    1 large glass of juice (20)
    1 cup cereal (10)
    2 slices toast (30)
    1 tablespoon sugar, honey, syrup, jam, or jelly (15)
Midmorning snack:
    20 g carbohydrate from list below (20)
Lunch:
    1–8 ounces soft drink (not sugar-free) (20)
    2 sandwiches (60)
    fruit, pie, or cake (20)
Midafternoon snack:
    20 g carbohydrate from lists below (20)
Dinner or supper:
    1 large glass juice (20)
    1 medium potato (20)
    1 serving vegetables (10); meat, salad, etc., as desired
    1 slice bread (15)
    1 serving ice cream (20)
Evening snack:
    Day 1 and 2 only; transfer 20 g carbohydrate from dinner or lunch.

List A (10 g carbohydrate)	List B (20 g carbohydrate)
1 slice bread	1 cup canned fruit
1 roll	1 ice cream soda
1 bun	8 ounces soft drink
1 muffin	4 filled cookies
1 plain doughnut	1 piece coffee cake
5 saltines	1 jelly doughnut
1 small pastry	8 ounces chocolate
1 piece fresh fruit (small)	1 piece pie
1 cup popcorn	1 piece iced cake
2 graham crackers	1 cup hot cereal
4 peanut butter nabs	1 cup macaroni
6 vanilla wafers	1 cup rice
8 ounces milk	1 cup spaghetti

Table 10–1 (continued)
Preparation for Oral Glucose Tolerance Test: 300-g Carbohydrate Diet

List A (10 g carbohydrate)	List B (20 g carbohydrate)
2 teaspoons sugar	1 cup noodles
1 small glass juice	2 pancakes
	1 cup ice cream
	1 cup pudding
	1 medium potato
	1 piece fresh fruit (large)
	½ cup corn

that carbohydrate tolerance deteriorates as a function of age.[17-19] Whether this indicates that the great bulk of the population, if they live to be old enough, will develop mild carbohydrate intolerance or whether this is merely a physiologic component of aging is still unclear. A widely used rule of thumb is to allow an additional 10 mg/dl increment for the upper limit of blood sugar for each decade of age over 50 years.

Diet, as previously mentioned, is probably the most important variable affecting glucose tolerance.

There are many factors involved in deciding on the optimal amount of physical activity to be allowed during the 3-day preparation period.[20,21] Probably the best approach is to keep physical activity for the 3 days prior to the test at the average level for that particular individual. It is also the author's opinion that no unusual amount of physical activity should be performed on the morning of the test (such as running or jogging). The amount of physical activity during the performance of the test itself should be limited. In the author's laboratory most patients sit quietly throughout the test, and some lie down for brief periods. A short walk to the lavatory is the maximum amount of activity allowed.

Table 10–2
Factors Influencing Glucose Tolerance

Diabetes heredity
Body weight
Age
Diet
Physical activity
Stress
Endocrine constellation
    Pituitary
    Thyroid
    Adrenals
Drugs
    Oral contraceptives
    Diuretics (thiazides)
    Anticonvulsants (diphenylhydantoin)
    Hormones (steroids)
Concomitant disease
    Neoplastic
    Nutritional
    Hepatic
    Debilitated states

Rather than make repeated venipunctures, we utilize an indwelling venous flexible plastic needle maintained patent by a saline infusion. Not only is this convenient for obtaining samples, it also minimizes the pain of repeated venipunctures and in addition tends to reduce the spontaneous physical activity of the testee.

It is probably wise not to test an individual at a time of transient stress. Deferring or postponing tests for young individuals so as not to be in conflict with scholastic examinations is warranted.

The general endocrine status of the patient should be kept in mind. If there are any clinical suspicions, suitable tests to rule out defects of the pituitary, thyroid, adrenals, or gonads should be done. In addition, a detailed drug history should be obtained prior to performing the test, and all optional medications that the individual is taking should be either temporarily omitted or postponed on the morning of the test day to reduce (as best as possible) interference of these materials with carbohydrate metabolism. It is clearly to be anticipated that drugs such as oral contraceptive agents, corticosteroids, thiazides, and diphenylhydantoin preparations might be responsible for mild carbohydrate intolerance.[22-24] It is also to be kept in mind that many individuals taking these compounds have normal glucose tolerance, despite the known effects of the drugs.

INTERPRETATION OF THE TEST IN AMBULATORY OUTPATIENTS

It is quite likely that use of the oral glucose tolerance test as part of an inpatient admission will lead to confusion in interpreting the results. If at all possible the test should be performed on an ambulatory outpatient basis. In addition, it must be kept in mind that concomitant disease (particularly neoplasia, debilitated states, chronic nutritional diseases, etc.) may have an important influence on the results.[25]

UPPER LIMITS OF NORMAL

It is known that whole blood glucose levels are about 15 percent lower than corresponding plasma glucose levels.[26] This is because glucose is soluble in the plasma water space and in the red cell water space, and removal of red cells (mostly hemoglobin) serves to increase the relative water space of the plasma sample as compared to the whole blood glucose sample.

Many different upper limits of normal have been suggested for the 100-g oral glucose tolerance test.[13] Table 10-3 shows some of the various criteria currently utilized in the United States; in general, they are quite similar. There has been a recent review[27] of some studies, apparently well controlled, that suggest deviations from the upper limits shown in this table. It is not clear, however, whether some of these studies have been influenced by one or more of the variables known to influence carbohydrate metabolism.

The establishment of so-called upper limits of normal tends to minimize in the minds of both patient and physician the fact that all biologic measurements have a very vague transition from true normality to true abnormality. The use of any single set of numbers always tends to imply a black–white, yes–no, good–bad juxtaposition, a single point of transition.

The author's laboratory has attempted to develop a sound data base with the 100-g

Table 10-3
Various Criteria for Upper Limits of Normal in Oral Glucose Tolerance Test

Group	Dose	Time (hr)					
		F	0.5	1	1.5	2	3
USPHS	100 g (Points)†	100* (1)	—	170 (1/2)	—	120 (1/2)	110 (1)
Joslin	100 g	100	—	160	—	120	110
Fajans/Conn	1.75 g/kg ideal body weight	—	—	160	140	120	—
Pregnancy (O'Sullivan)	100 g	90	—	165	—	145	125

*All values are venous whole blood glucose, milligrams per deciliter.
†One or more points = diabetes.

Implications from Oral Glucose Tolerance

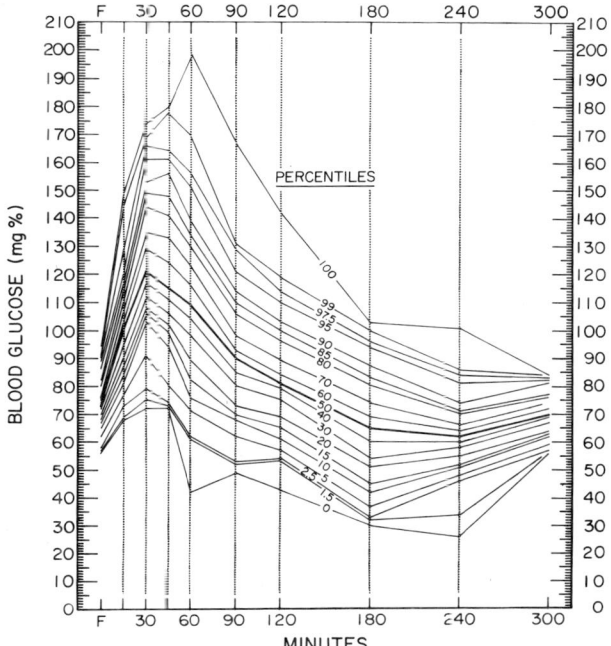

Fig. 10-1. Blood glucose percentiles computed from data available on 135 males, nonobese, ages 15-44 years.

oral glucose tolerance test in relatively young nonobese individuals. Over 100 male and 100 female subjects, with no known family history of diabetes, between the ages of 15 and 44 years have been evaluated under standard testing conditions. In addition to calculation of an absolute blood sugar level as the upper limit of normal at the various time intervals studied, it has been possible to take the blood glucose data (for the males and the females separately) and perform a distribution analysis so that a percentile can be calculated for each glucose level at each time interval during the oral glucose tolerance test. In this fashion any test in a study subject can be assessed not in terms of whether the value exceeds or does not exceed any upper limit of normal but in terms of whether the value falls at or near various percentile ranks seen in a comparable normal control population. A similar approach for glucose tolerance in children has been advocated.[28]

Figure 10-1 shows the distribution of percentiles for the data accumulated in oral glucose tolerance tests performed on 135 healthy, normal male controls. The time intervals of the test from the fasting sample to the 300-min sample are shown in the lower and upper horizontal margins of the figure, and whole blood glucose levels (obtained by AutoAnalyzer ferricyanide method) are shown at both left and right vertical margins. Thus any blood glucose level at any time interval can be appropriately evaluated by laying a straightedge to connect the glucose levels on the right and left margins and converting to one of the nearest percentile ranks on the basis of the curves in the figure. The actual percentiles are shown for the decile and some intermediate intervals. Figure 10-2 shows a similar display of the data accumulated in 110 normal female controls.

One may ask why the sexes are separated. A comparison of the two figures will show that there is a clinically meaningful significant difference between the distributions of

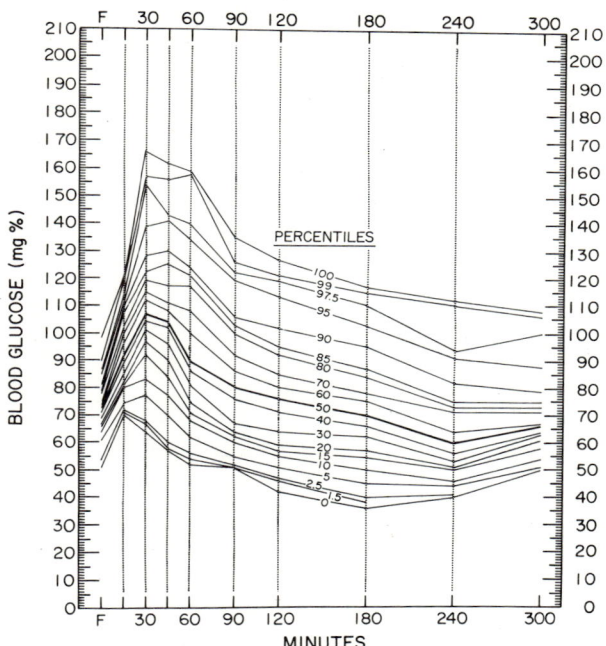

Fig. 10-2. Blood glucose percentiles calculated from 110 females, nonobese, ages 15-44.

blood glucose levels of the males and the females. Parenthetically it can be stated that there are a number of time intervals during which the mean blood glucose levels are significantly different for the two sexes. For the purposes at hand, both the upper limits and the lower limits at certain important percentile levels are clearly different for the two sexes.

A few illustrations will indicate how these figures can be utilized. If one wishes to interpret a blood glucose level of 160 mg/dl at the 1-hr time interval in a nonobese male who is between the ages of 15 and 44 years, it can be seen that this falls between percentiles 97.5 and 99. This would clearly be a highly suspicious glucose level. If a similar individual at the 1-hr time interval has a blood glucose level of 150 mg/dl, this would appear to be reassuring in that it is 10 mg/dl lower than that deemed to be clinically meaningful, but it can be seen that this is approximately at the 95 percentile rank and is probably not that much "biologically" significantly lower than the level of 160 mg/dl of the first man.

In regard to patients suspected of having reactive hypoglycemia, it can be seen that among females approximately 10 percent of the population tested had blood sugar levels below 50 mg/dl at the 3-hr time interval. Only 2.5 percent of the population had levels below approximately 40 mg/dl, and the clear-cut lower limit (0 percentile) was approximately 36 mg/dl. Among males, nearly 15 percent of the population showed blood sugar levels equal to or lower than 50 mg/dl at 180 min, and the absolute lower limit was nearer 30 mg/dl.

Thus it is suggested that not the upper and lower limits of normal but the ranking by percentile is important in assessing the glucose level achieved by a patient, as this can

Table 10-4
Comparison of Patterns Abnormality (Ab) and Normality (N) during a Standard Oral Glucose Tolerance Test (OGTT) and a Cortisone-primed Oral Glucose Tolerance Test (COGTT) in Offspring of Conjugal Diabetics*

Pattern	Number	Percentage
N–OGTT N–COGTT	67	72
N–OGTT Ab–COGTT	6 ⎱ $p < 0.02$	7.5
Ab–OGTT N–COGTT	15 ⎰	16
Ab–OGTT Ab–COGTT	5	5.5

*$n = 93$; ages 15–49 years; nonobese

allow a better perspective on the degree of normality or abnormality of that level. A plasma glucose level can be converted (approximately) to a whole blood glucose level by multiplying by 0.85.

PRIOR STEROID ADMINISTRATION

In the hope that the cortisone-primed oral glucose tolerance test, as suggested by Fajans and Conn,[6] might provide data more useful than the standard oral glucose tolerance test in an ambulatory outpatient setting, a number of normal control males and females were tested by both methods. Since the normal subjects who had cortisone-primed tests (males and females separated) were fewer than 100 (not sufficient for distributional analysis), the upper limit of normal was chosen as the mean plus two standard deviations at each time interval for each type of test. Slight adjustment factors of very small magnitude were used, so that assessment of the performances of these same normals by these criteria showed that approximately 2.5 percent of the normal males and normal females were judged abnormal during the cortisone-primed oral glucose tolerance test and the standard test.

Both the oral glucose tolerance test and the cortisone-primed test were then performed in random order in a population selected on genetic grounds to have a high probability of having carbohydrate intolerance.

As seen in Table 10-4, significantly more offspring (not known to have diabetes) of two diabetic parents were found who had abnormal oral tests and normal cortisone-primed tests than offspring who had abnormal cortisone-primed tests and normal oral tests. Therefore, in this outpatient ambulatory testing facility and with the population under study, it was concluded that the cortisone-primed test was not more sensitive than the standard oral glucose tolerance test.

THE MEANING OF MILDLY ABNORMAL RESULTS

It has been difficult to quantify the degree of reproducibility of the standard oral glucose tolerance test, particularly over long periods of time in follow-up studies of the same subjects. Some studies have suggested a reasonable degree of reproducibility for the test, and others have found that the oral glucose tolerance test is not very reproducible. But perhaps of more clinical importance is how often one encounters an abnormal test, as judged by reasonable criteria, in an individual who previously had a normal test, and vice versa. To evaluate the clinical meaning of small degrees of abnormality of the oral test, repeated tests were performed 1–2 years apart in a number of offspring of two diabetic parents. These individuals had no clinical symptoms or signs suggestive of diabetes. The upper limits of normal for the oral glucose tolerance test were identical to those used in the previous study that compared the standard oral test to the cortisone-primed test.

It can be seen in Figure 10–3 that 67 offspring of two diabetic parents were studied. The subjects were between the ages of 10 and 50 years and were nonobese. An analysis of the first oral glucose tolerance test in these 67 subjects showed that 23 (34 percent) were abnormal (chemical diabetics). The degree of abnormality seen was relatively mild, usually consisting in a normal fasting blood glucose value, with one or two postglucose values elevated. The results of the test were reported to all individuals, and in those in whom the test was deemed abnormal it was indicated that the degree of abnormality was not alarming. No diet or drug therapy was utilized in these subjects. In 1–2 years the test was repeated under identical circumstances, and it can be seen that 18 of the 67 subjects showed abnormality (27 percent). It is clear, however, that the distribution of the abnormal tests was different on the second test as compared to the first. Nine patients who previously had normal tests manifested abnormal results on their second tests, while 35 individuals showed continuing normal results. If the criterion used to define an individual as a chemical diabetic is taken to be the presence of one or more abnormal test results in a series of tests, it can be seen that 48 percent of the subjects could be termed chemical diabetics.

The test was repeated a third time after an additional 1–2 years, and the results show that 25 percent of these third tests were abnormal, with the number of chemical diabetics increasing to 55 percent. It can also be seen that there is random occurrence of normal and abnormal test results on repeated tests in this group, with no definite pattern emerging.

An attempt was made to study in a similar manner a group of normal healthy volunteers with no family history of diabetes. This proved extremely difficult; however, 19 such subjects have been studied in parallel with the 67 offspring of two diabetic parents, and the results are shown in Figure 10–4. It can be seen that in only 1 subject at one test (the second test) was there an abnormal result.

A number of conclusions can be drawn. First, the specific upper limits of normal that were chosen appear to be neither too liberal nor too conservative, since in the normal control population the anticipated false positive test rate of 2 percent was seen. Second, the clinical implications of a chemical diabetic oral glucose tolerance test and the value of a single standard oral glucose tolerance test in detecting early carbohydrate intolerance must be questioned. In 9 patients (13 percent) abnormal tests were followed by abnormal tests. In 14 patients (21 percent) abnormal tests were followed by normal tests. But in 9 patients normal tests were followed by abnormal tests (13 percent), and in 35 offspring normal tests were followed by normal tests (52 percent). This might suggest either that the offspring of two diabetic parents fluctuate in and out of mild carbohydrate intolerance or

Implications from Oral Glucose Tolerance

TEST	NO. OF ABNORMAL TESTS	NO. OF OFFSPRING (Abnormal and Normal Tests)								NO. OF CHEMICAL DIABETICS
		7	2	4	10	1	8	5	30	
# 1	23/67 (34%)	Ab	Ab	Ab	Ab	N	N	N	N	23/67 (34%)
# 2	18/67 (27%)	Ab	Ab	N	N	Ab	Ab	N	N	32/67 (48%)
# 3	17/67 (25%)	Ab	N	Ab	N	Ab	N	Ab	N	37/67 (55%)
Total =	58/201 (29%)							Total =		37/67 (55%)

Fig. 10–3. Patterns of abnormality and normality seen over the course of three oral glucose tolerance tests performed 1–2 years apart. Data obtained from 67 offspring of two diabetic parents, ages 10–50 years, weight less than 121 percent of ideal body weight.

that the test reproducibility is poor and allows for no clinical interpretation. It is probably unwarranted to attribute much clinical significance to a single chemical diabetic test; it is possible that only repeated testing will provide definitive information. One should be very cautious about applying the label diabetes mellitus to an individual on the basis of a single chemical diabetic test. Important implications regarding insurability or employment must be taken into consideration.

Smaller numbers of study subjects (offspring of two diabetic parents) have been studied over longer periods of time with repeated oral glucose testing. Figure 10–5 summarizes the results in progressively smaller groups who have had from 3 to 6 repeated tests. The percentages of detected chemical diabetics are plotted in relationship to the number of repeat oral glucose tolerance tests. It can be seen that with each additional testing additional numbers of offspring of two diabetic parents who previously had normal tests show abnormalities. Eventually, after multiple repeated testing, between 70 and 80 percent of the individuals have shown at least one abnormal test in the series. These intermittent abnormal tests do not appear to show any sex differences and do not appear to be related to the age of the subject. Currently under investigation are the questions

TEST	NO. OF ABNORMAL TESTS	NO. OF NORMALS (Abnormal and Normal Tests)								NO. OF CHEMICAL DIABETICS
		0	0	0	0	0	1	0	18	
# 1	0/19 (0%)	Ab	Ab	Ab	Ab	N	N	N	N	0/19 (0%)
# 2	1/19 (5%)	Ab	Ab	N	N	Ab	Ab	N	N	1/19 (5%)
# 3	0/19 (0%)	Ab	N	Ab	N	Ab	N	Ab	N	1/19 (5%)
Total =	1/57 (2%)							Total =		1/19 (5%)

Fig. 10–4. Patterns of abnormality and normality seen over the course of three oral glucose tolerance tests performed 1–2 years apart. Data obtained from 19 normal controls with no known family history of diabetes, ages 10–50 years, weight less than 121 percent of ideal body weight.

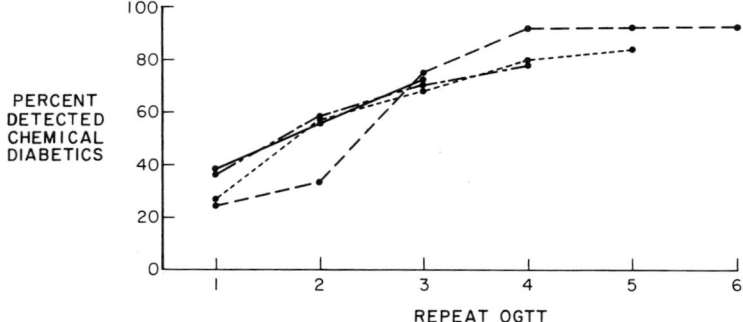

Fig. 10–5. Percentage detected chemical diabetics in the population of offspring of two diabetic parents who have had repeated oral glucose tolerance tests (OGTT) 1–2 years apart. Data are shown for those individuals who have had either 3, 4, 5, or 6 completed standard oral glucose tolerance tests.

whether there is any evidence that this intermittent carbohydrate intolerance is present at even a very young age, whether there are any significant metabolic or structural abnormalities associated with chemical diabetes, and how often these chemical diabetics progress to clinical diabetes.

INCREASE IN GLUCOSE INTOLERANCE IN HIGH-RISK PATIENTS

The previous data were concerned only with whether the results of the tests were normal or abnormal. Other analyses of this population have been made to see whether there is any evidence of a progressive but slow deterioration in glucose tolerance. Figure 10–6 compares the mean blood glucose levels achieved during oral glucose tolerance tests in 24 offspring of two diabetic parents, comparing their initial tests to follow-up tests that were performed 5–8 years after the initial tests. It can be seen that the mean levels are very similar and that, if anything, lower levels are seen on the follow-up tests. Thus there is no evidence of any progressive deterioration in the overall carbohydrate tolerance of this group over the observed period. It is speculated that a large fraction of these offspring may exhibit only a mild degree of nonprogressive intermittent chemical diabetes.

DIABETES DIATHESIS IN OFFSPRING OF TWO DIABETIC PARENTS

The oral glucose tolerance test has provided important information in such families. The following estimates are based on 10 years of experience in evaluating approximately 300 offspring of two diabetic parents from approximately 120 families. In only a small

Implications from Oral Glucose Tolerance

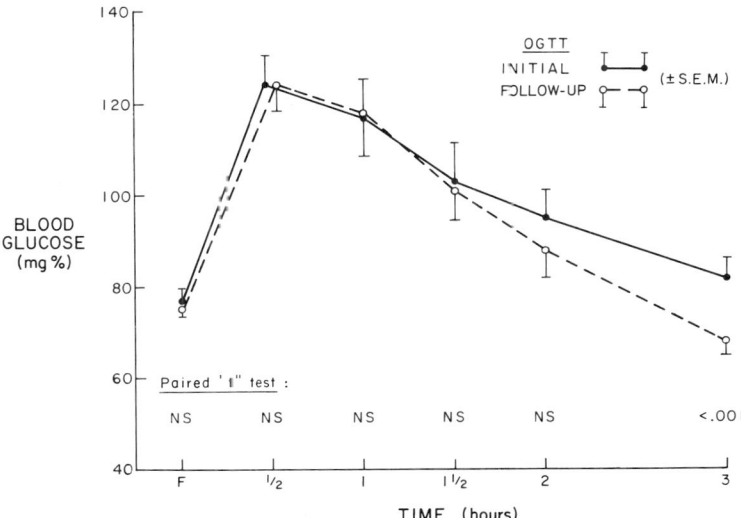

Fig. 10-6. Comparison of mean blood glucose levels during the course of an initial oral glucose tolerance test and a follow-up oral glucose tolerance test performed 5 years or more after the initial test. Data obtained from 24 offspring of two diabetic parents.

fraction of these families (about 10 percent) did one of the two parents have the juvenile form of disease. It is clear from numerous recent studies that juvenile diabetes may be less heritable than maturity-onset diabetes, but in this current estimate all families have been included to provide an overview.

At the time such families are identified (soon after development of diabetes in the second parent), approximately 2 percent of their offspring will already have juvenile-type insulin-dependent diabetes.

Detailed evaluation of medical records on additional known diabetic offspring suggests that at the time of identification of these families approximately 15 percent of offspring have the maturity-onset form of the disease. An additional 2 percent appear to have a milder maturity form of the disease that can be treated by diet restriction. From the results in the families that were studied for 10 years, it can be estimated that a very small fraction of these individuals develop symptomatic diabetes during this period. Making crude estimations of what might happen as this population ages to approximately 85 years, the data suggest that approximately 25-35 percent will develop overt diabetes.

Multiple glucose tolerance testing suggests that of the remaining offspring about 70-80 percent will develop intermittent chemical diabetes. It is also estimated that about 10 to 13 percent will remain nondiabetic and continuously glucose-tolerant.

Table 10-5
Estimates of Risk of Developing Diabetes

Group	1965	1975
Offspring of conjugal Diabetics	100%	35% overt 50% chemical 15% nondiabetic

Table 10–5 indicates how estimates have changed over the past 10 years in regard to anticipated development of diabetes in this high-risk group.

TESTING IN SO-CALLED REACTIVE HYPOGLYCEMIA

It has become clear, particularly over the past 10 years, that some individuals apparently have a metabolic defect that leads to repetitive occurrences of one or more signs and symptoms that are associated with hypoglycemia. These symptoms occur 2–4 hr after ingestion of a meal, and they are of sufficient frequency and intensity to lead the individual to seek medical assistance. The symptom constellation is diffuse and nonspecific. It may include irritability, sweatinesss, tingling of the hands, difficulty with vision, headache, inability to concentrate, dizziness, etc. On oral glucose tolerance testing the individual's specific clinical constellation of symptoms is dramatically reproduced, and a large percentage of these individuals show blood sugar levels below 50 mg/dl between 2 and 5 hr after oral glucose administration. As discussed previously, this commonly used lower limit of normal for the oral glucose tolerance test does not agree with the distributions of blood glucose levels in normal individuals similarly tested. Thus the terms symptomatic reactive hypoglycemia and biochemical reactive hypoglycemia might be utilized.

A number of subjects presenting with the previous described symptoms have been evaluated by the oral glucose tolerance test in the author's laboratory and compared not only with normal control subjects but also with groups of prediabetics (offspring of two diabetic parents) and with groups of nonobese and obese offspring who have abnormal glucose tolerance tests (chemical diabetics).

Table 10–6 shows the distribution of blood glucose levels lower than 51 mg/dl during the oral glucose tolerance test. It can be seen that there is no significant difference in the distributions of these blood sugar levels among the groups.

Table 10–7 compares the mean levels of blood glucose during oral glucose tolerance testing in the normal controls and in the 13 patients with symptomatic reactive hypoglycemia. It can be seen that during the first hour after glucose administration the patients with reactive hypoglycemia have blood glucose levels lower than those seen in the normal controls, but during the latter portion of the test the blood glucose levels are not significantly different, despite the appearance of the patient's symptom complex.

Insulin levels show no significant differences between the mean levels seen in the normal controls and the levels in the patients with reactive hypoglycemia. The pattern of insulin release, however, does seem different in the patients with reactive hypoglycemia, and as shown in Table 10–7, the patients with reactive hypoglycemia show significantly earlier peaks and significantly greater insulinogenic indices than do the normal controls.

A percentage of the patients with reactive hypoglycemia exhibit cerebral symptomatology and adenergic responses suggestive of hypoglycemia, but at glucose levels that are within the normal range (although on the lower end). The evidence seen thus far suggests an extraordinarily brisk beta cell response (enhanced early phase of insulin secretion?). An inappropriate elevation of the level of insulin in comparison to the degree of glycemic stimulus is also noted. One can postulate that translocation of glucose from vascular space into central nervous system tissues might be impaired in these individuals, so that they experience neuroglycopenia and its resultant symptoms at blood glucose levels that are not unduly low.

Table 10-6
Incidence of Postoral Glucose "Hypoglycemia"

Group	(n)	Percentages (and Numbers) with Venous Blood Glucose (mg/dl) Equal to or Less than				
		50	45	40	35	30
Controls	(123)	23(29)*	11(14)	6(7)	2(3)	0
Prediabetics	(84)	25(21)	17(14)	5(4)	1(1)	0
Chemical diabetics	(42)	14(6)	2(1)	0(0)	0(0)	0
Chemical diabetics, obese	(18)	22(4)	17(3)	6(1)	0(0)	0
Symptomatic hypoglycemics	(13)	39(5)	31(4)	0(0)	0(0)	0

*Percentage, followed by number of patients in parentheses.

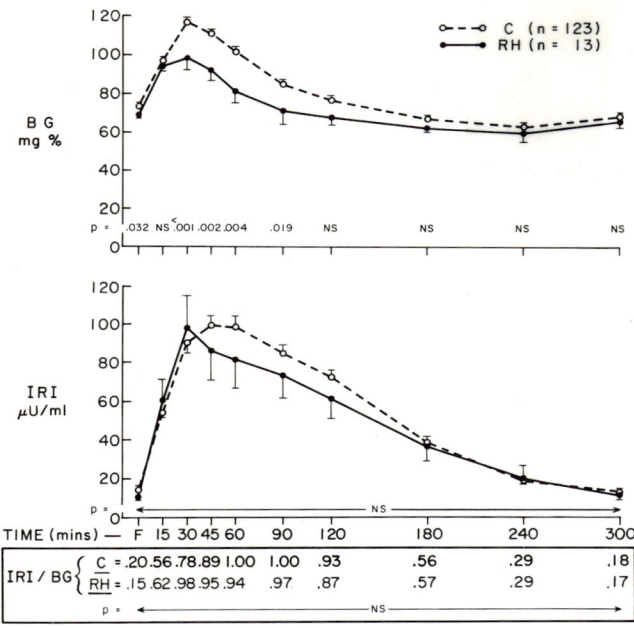

Fig. 10–7. Mean levels of blood glucose (BG) and serum insulin (IRI) during oral glucose tolerance testing in normal controls (C) and in patients with reactive hypoglycemia (RH). Also shown is the insulin blood glucose ratio computed at each time interval. Pertinent statistical differences are shown.

Table 10-7
IRI-BG Relationship during OGTT in Reactive Hypoglycemics and Controls

	Controls	Reactive Hypoglycemics	p
Age (years)	26.60 ± 0.58*	28.08 ± 1.80*	n.s.
Ideal weight (%)	99.80 ± 0.83	91.14 ± 3.48	0.019
Peak IRI (μU/ml)	121.33 ± 5.83	120.85 ± 13.39	n.s.
Time of peak IRI (min)	60.61 ± 2.81	40.38 ± 5.73	0.024
0-60 BG area (mg% x min)	1823 ± 67	1228 ± 186	0.007
0-60 IRI area (μU/ml x min)	3660 ± 185	3828 ± 594	n.s.
0-60 IRI/BG	2.30 ± 0.15	4.30 ± 1.27	0.002
0-300 BG area (mg% x min)	3242 ± 152	2324 ± 579	n.s
0-300 IRI area (μU/ml x min)	11416 ± 507	11344 ± 1588	n.s.
0-300 IRI/BG	4.68 ± 0.37	8.62 ± 2.46	0.010
"b" (μU/ml per mg%)	1.36 ± 0.07	1.55 ± 0.33	n.s.

*Mean ± SEM.

CONCLUSIONS AND SUMMARY

The oral glucose tolerance test, although imperfect, is still the mainstay in diagnosis of early carbohydrate tolerance; in addition, it has been a valuable tool in a variety of investigative studies focused on the pathogenesis of diabetes mellitus. Attempts must be made to provide a better test for this purpose; there have been many attempts over the years, but no test has yet supplanted the oral glucose tolerance test. It is suggested that great care be taken in preparing the patient for the test; there are many variables that can alter the test result and as many as possible should be eliminated. The test has also been useful in clarifying some confusing problems in patients with idiopathic reactive hypoglycemia.

REFERENCES

1. Jacobsen A: Untersuchungen über den Einfluss des Chloralhydrats auf experimentelle Hyperglykamieformen. Biochem Z 51:443, 1913 1913
2. Forster H, Haslbeck M, Mehnert H: Metabolic studies following the oral ingestion of different doses of glucose. Diabetes 21:1102, 1972
3. Exton WG, Rose AR: A one-hour two dose glucose tolerance test based on Allen's paradoxical law. Am J Clin Pathol 4:381, 1934
4. Steinke J, Soeldner JS, Camerini-Davalos, et al: Studies on serum insulin-like activity (ILA) in prediabetes and early overt diabetes. Diabetes 12:502, 1963
5. Bowen AJ, Reeves RL: Diurnal variation in glucose tolerance. Arch Intern Med 119:261, 1967
6. Fajans SS, Conn JW: An approach to the prediction of diabetes mellitus by modification of the glucose tolerance test with cortisone. Diabetes 3:296, 1954
7. Ikkos D, Luft R: On the intravenous glucose tolerance test. Acta Endocrinol 25:312, 1957
8. Kahn CB, Soeldner JS, Gleason RE, et al: Clinical and chemical diabetes in offspring of diabetic couples. N Engl J Med 281:343, 1969
9. Nadon GW, Little JA, Hall WE, et al: A comparison of the oral and the intravenous glucose tolerance tests in the nondiabetic, possible diabetic and diabetic subjects. Can Med Assoc J 91:1350, 1964
10. Olefsky JM, Farquhar JW, Reaven GM: Do the oral and intravenous glucose tolerance tests provide similar diagnostic information in patients with chemical diabetes mellitus? Diabetes 22:202, 1973
11. Leonards JR, McCullagh EP, Christopher TC: A new carbohydrate solution for testing glucose tolerance. Diabetes 14:96, 1965
12. Unger RH, Madison LL: Comparison of response to intravenously administered sodium tolbutamide in mild diabetic and nondiabetic subjects. J Clin Invest 37:627, 1958
13. Klimt CR, Prout TE, Bradley RF, et al: Standardizations of the oral glucose tolerance test (report of the Committee on Statistics of the American Diabetes Association, June 14, 1968). Diabetes 18:299, 1969
14. Conn JW: Interpretation of the glucose tolerance test. The necessity of a standard preparatory diet. Am J Med Sci 199:555, 1940
15. Wilkerson HLC, Butler FK, Francis JO: The effect of prior carbohydrate intake on the oral glucose tolerance test. Diabetes 9:386, 1960
16. Paullin JE, Sauls HC: A study of the glucose tolerance test in the obese. South Med J 15:249, 1922
17. Brandt RL: Decreased carbohydrate tolerance in elderly patients. Geriatrics 15:315, 1960
18. Streeten DHP, Gerstein MM, Marmor BM, et al: Reduced glucose tolerance in elderly human subjects. Diabetes 14:579, 1965
19. Pozefsky T, Colker JL, Langs HM, et al: The cortisone-glucose tolerance test. The influence of age on performance. Ann Intern Med 63:988, 1965
20. Blotner H: Effect of prolonged physical inactivity on tolerance of sugar. Arch Intern Med 75:39, 1945
21. Lipman RL, Raskin P, Love T, et al: Glucose intolerance during decreased physical activity in man. Diabetes 21:101, 1972
22. Wynn V, Doar JWH: Some effects of oral contraceptives on carbohydrate metabolism. Lancet 2:715, 1966
23. Rapoport MI, Hurd HF: Thiazide-induced glucose intolerance treated with potassium. Arch Intern Med 113:405, 1964
24. Peters BH, Samaan NA: Hyperglycemia with relative hypoinsulinemia in diphenylhydantoin toxicity. N Engl J Med 281:91, 1969

25. Hecht A, Weisenfeld S, Goldner MG: Factors influencing oral glucose tolerance: Experience with chronically ill patients. Metabolism 10:712, 1961
26. Zalme E, Knowles HC Jr: A plea for plasma sugar. Diabetes 14:165, 1965
27. Siperstein MD: The glucose tolerance test: A pitfall in the diagnosis of diabetes mellitus. Adv Intern Med 20:297, 1975
28. Jackson RL, Guthrie RA: The Child with Diabetes Mellitus, Current Concepts Series. Kalamazoo, Upjohn, 1975

Thaddeus E. Prout

11
The Prudent Physician

For over 7 years members of the medical community concerned with the care of patients with diabetes have been unable to escape the debate over the relative merits of the various current methods of treatment of maturity-onset diabetes mellitus. The original report of the University Group Diabetes Program (UGDP)[1-3] on the effects of oral hypoglycemic drugs, discussions of the report's clinical implications,[4,5] criticisms con[6] and pro,[7] and independent reviews of the scientific merits of the study[8-10] are principal references in this debate.

There is actually a great deal of common ground involved in the current forms of therapy of these patients that is not controversial. There are also areas in which the present evidence, although not conclusive, is strongly in favor of one form of therapy over another under the ancient dictum *primum nocere*. Thus areas of debate that are unresolved are minor. The present status of therapy of the diabetic should therefore be summarized for the prudent physician who wishes, above all, to give his patients the best available care.

Calorie control and/or body weight control are the first principles of therapy of the diabetic patient. Normalization of plasma glucose, cholesterol, and triglyceride may be attained through dietary therapy, even when normal body weight is not attained.[11] Normalization of these risk factors would be facilitated by better methods of dietary instruction and longer periods of dietary therapy than are now generally available in most communities. Although not all physicians are fully convinced that plasma glucose and lipid control can in most instances be achieved by vigorous dietary effort or that such normalization of these factors necessarily prevents the complications of diabetes, it is generally agreed that these are reasonable therapeutic goals[12] and that they should be pursued more vigorously than they have been in the recent past.

Oral agents in general have been used uncritically in the past. They are contraindicated in patients in whom they do not have any significant pharmacologic effect on plasma glucose. The practice of continuing their use without evidence of efficacy ("primary and secondary failure") and without retesting for continued need in patients who have attained control of plasma glucose (by trial for a period on diet alone) violates the cardinal principle of not using any drug without evidence of benefit. It is apparently not widely appreciated that in a great many patients the effects of these drugs in lowering plasma glucose levels may be only temporary.

Phenformin has now been associated with increases in the overall death rate, the cardiovascular death rate, and the incidence of hypertension.[3] Ancillary findings of increased pulse rates, increased angina, increased necessity for use of digitalis preparations and hypotensive agents, and increased hospitalization rates give additional evidence that patients treated with phenformin do less well than do patients treated with insulin or diet alone. No acute or chronic benefit can be attributed to phenformin use.[10]

There is no study that has demonstrated that the combination of sulfonylureas and phenformin, within the limits of recommended dosage, is effective when neither is effective alone. It should be readily agreed on by all concerned that there is no virtue in increasing the risks by having patients take additional noneffective drugs.

Every death due to lactic acidosis in association with phenformin therapy implicates phenformin as a possible cause.[12] Lactic acidosis complicated by phenformin therapy is a highly lethal disease; it is entirely unlike the milder degrees of lactic acidosis found in association with even profound degrees of oxygen desaturation in patients not on phenformin. We have hidden too long behind statements implying that lactic acidosis is a complicated condition brought on by the patient's circumstances and that phenformin, when present, can rarely be blamed.

As to the sulfonylureas, although only one drug was used in the clinical trials carried out in the UGDP, it is prudent from a safety standpoint to consider that the results found *may* also apply to other hypoglycemic agents in this class, although this remains unproven. This is particularly true in view of the close similarities that have been found among the modes of action of all the sulfonylurea drugs tested thus far, as well as their chemical similarities.[13] This is not to say that the detrimental effects found for tolbutamide could not be due to a metabolite of this specific drug, but it strongly implies, in the absence of any greater benefit than has thus far been shown, that members of the sulfonylurea family should be employed with far more caution than in the past.[14]

It should be accepted that the sulfonylureas are contraindicated in patients who have shown serious hypoglycemic reactions to sulfonylurea drugs. Among the reported cases collected by Seltzer,[15] between one-fifth and one-sixth of the patients who were listed as having had hypoglycemic reactions in association with oral drugs had died. This evidence was accumulated after a decade of use of these drugs; moreover, they were used by practitioners who had optimal experience in their administration. On the basis of this experience, it would again seem prudent to avoid use of these agents in the older age group, since they have been found to be susceptible to serious hypoglycemic action and since no specific benefit can be expected. It would be imprudent in the extreme to place even more powerful new drugs of this class on the market and run an even greater risk of this danger in other patients. Tolbutamide is, according to all available comparisons, the safest sulfonylurea drug. It is better to "bear those ills we have than to fly to others that we know not of."[16] Moreover, tolbutamide, which is now available as a generic drug, is far less expensive for our patients.

There is evidence, not only in the UGDP study but in other studies as well, of increased jeopardy for patients with coronary heart disease who have episodes of myocardial ischemia while on sulfonylurea drugs. The findings of increased case fatality rates in the UGDP,[2] increased myocardial irritability,[13] and increased deaths from ventricular fibrillation for patients on sulfonylureas when compared to patients on insulin or diet[17] should lead us to conclude that patients have less chance of survival with the occurrence of an acute myocardial insult if they are on sulfonylurea drugs. If one wishes to argue that this is not conclusively proven, it is well to remember that one can find scant evidence for beneficial effect; once again, prudence should determine against a risk that is unwarranted. In this context we should all be agreed that use of all sulfonylurea drugs is contraindicated in patients with coronary heart disease at risk of a myocardial event.[14]

Finally, there is the matter of the patients' understanding of what is at stake when they begin to take or elect to continue to take oral hypoglycemic agents. In view of the possible risks associated with use of these drugs and the virtual absence of any benefit other than their convenience, patients should participate in the decision to use these drugs based on information that is timely and complete. It should be emphasized at the time of that decision and at subsequent interviews that the drug should be withdrawn at the earliest sign of any potential problem.

If these be the areas of agreement, where are the areas of dissent and disagreement? Interestingly enough, the disagreement appears to be in the details rather than in the general principles.

First, there may be disagreement as to how long one should pursue the trail of diet alone and tolerate hyperglycemia before introducing a therapeutic agent to lower the plasma glucose. Just how important it is to maintain normal plasma glucose is somewhat uncertain, since there is little evidence in the reported findings of the UGDP study to suggest that untoward effects are any greater among patients with adult-onset diabetes treated with diet alone than among those on various quantities of insulin designated to normalize circulating levels of glucose. It should be recalled that the latter group had a mandatory increase in insulin either for a fasting whole blood glucose over 110 mg/dl or for a whole blood glucose over 210 mg/dl drawn 1 hr after glucose challenge. Although with further observations this may not prove to be true for the lifetime of the diabetic patient, it is clearly more important to reduce total body weight and caloric intake over a prolonged period of time than to react too quickly to hyperglycemia and lose the opportunity to inculcate good principles of total care at the onset. Indeed, it is not clearly prudent to lower blood glucose by driving excess calories into fat stores and atherogenic plaques, as has been done heretofore.[18]

Second, there may be some disagreement over what constitutes secondary failure. Some definitions of secondary failure would lead physicians interested in tight control to take the same patients off oral agents as would those physicians who adhere to the lessons taught by the UGDP. In the first instance, physicians who believe that all diabetics should have postprandial blood glucose determinations of less than 150 mg/dl will find these agents extremely ineffecitve in a large majority of patients. To those who understand and accept the conclusions of the UGDP, these same patients will be taken off oral agents because the benefits are not visible and because diet is safer and more effective when properly followed.[11]

The major area of disagreement concerns a very small group of patients who successfully follow their diet and reduce their body weight but who continue to have glucose determinations above the levels that their individual physicians believe to be in their best interests and who, in addition, are known to be responsive to sulfonylurea agents. Physicians who are greatly concerned about the level of blood glucose will wish to have this level of blood glucose lowered. It is preferable to do this with insulin because it is universally effective, and the UGDP study suggests that it is safer.

Physicians and their patients in this group who wish to take the added overall increased risk of 1 percent per year found in the UGDP study should heed the warnings inherent in presently available evidence, and they should be very reluctant to continue the use of sulfonylureas in the presence of known coronary heart disease. The prudent physician, after judging the relative merits of phenformin therapy on the basis of current evidence, will have difficulty in justifying continued use of this drug in diabetic patients under any circumstances.[10]

REFERENCES

1. University Group Diabetes Program: A study of the effects of hypoglycemic agents on vascular complications in patients with adult-onset diabetes. I. Design, methods and baseline results. Diabetes 19 [Suppl 19]: 747–783, 1970.
2. University Group Diabetes Program: A study of the effects of hypoglycemic agents on vascular complications in patients with adult-onset diabetes. II. Mortality results. Diabetes 19 [Suppl 19]: 789–830, 1970.
3. University Group Diabetes Program: A study of the effects of hypoglycemic agents on vascular complications in patients with adult-onset diabetes. V. Evaluation of phenformin therapy. Diabetes 24 [Suppl I]: 65–184, 1975
4. University Group Diabetes Program: A study of the effects of hypoglycemic agents on vascular complications in patients with adult-onset diabetes. III. Clinical implications of UGDP results. JAMA 218:1400–1410, 1971
5. Prout TE: A prospective view of the treatment of adult-onset diabetes; with special reference to the University Group Diabetes Program and oral hypoglycemic agents. Med Clin North Am 55:1065–1076, 1971
6. Seltzer HS: A summary of criticisms of the findings and conclusions of the University Group Diabetes Program (UGDP). Diabetes 21:976–979, 1972
7. University Group Diabetes Program: The UGDP controversy: clinical trials versus clinical impressions. Diabetes 21:1035–1040, 1972
8. Report of the Committee for the Assessment of the Biometric Aspects of Controlled Trials of Hypoglycemic Agents. JAMA 231:583, 1975
9. Bradley RF, Dolger H, Forsham PH, et al: Settling the UGDP controversy? JAMA 232:813–817, 1975
10. Williams RH, Palmer JP: Farewell to phenformin for treating diabetes mellitus. Ann Intern Med 83:567, 1975
11. Davidson JK: The FDA and hypoglycemic drugs. JAMA 232:853, 1975
12. Winegrad AI, Clements, RS Jr, Morrison AD: Oral antidiabetic agents have a limited place in management and may be harmful, in Ingelfinger FJ, Ebert RV, Finland M, et al (eds): Controversy in Internal Medicine, vol II. Philadelphia, WB Saunders, 1974, pp 389–403
13. Levey GS, Lasseter KC, Palmer RF: Ann Rev Med 25:389, 1974
14. Freeman RB, Smith WMcF, Richardson JA, et al: Long-term therapy for chronic bacteiuria in men. Ann Intern Med 83–143, 1975
15. Seltzer HS: Drug induced hypoglycemia: A review based on 473 cases. Diabetes 21:955, 1972
16. Shakespeare W: Hamlet, act 3, sc 1
17. Soler NG, Pentecost BL, Bennet MH, et al: Coronary care for myocardial infarction in diabetes. Lancet 1:475, 1974
18. Wu CF, Haider B, Ahmed SS, et al: The effects of Tolbutamide on the Myocardium in Experimental Diabetes. Circulation 55:200, 1977

Philip Felig

12
Pathophysiology and Treatment of Diabetic Ketoacidosis

Diabetic ketoacidosis (DKA) is an acute, life-threatening medical emergency requiring rapid diagnosis and institution of proper treatment. Since the advent of insulin therapy over 50 years ago, the importance of DKA as a cause of death in the diabetic population has progressively declined. Nevertheless, this condition continues to be characterized by a mortality rate of 5–15 percent. Despite our long and generally successful experience in the management of this disorder, it is only in the last 5 years that much of our understanding of its pathogenesis has been unraveled. Furthermore, new recommendations (e.g., low-dose insulin), as well as some degree of controversy, characterize the approach to management of DKA.

PATHOGENESIS

DKA develops as a consequence of an absolute or relative deficiency of insulin that may result from failure of endogenous insulin secretion (as in the newly discoverd diabetic), from inadequate administration of exogenous insulin (in the known, insulin-dependent diabetic), or from increased requirements for insulin engendered by the stress associated with an intercurrent infectious, inflammatory, traumatic, or endocrinologic disorder. The increased insulin requirements in such disorders may be attributed to augmented secretion of hormones that have actions antagonistic to insulin (i.e., epinephrine, cortisol, glucagon, and growth hormone). Insulin deficiency results in abnormalities in carbohydrate, fat, and protein metabolism that pose a threat to the patient's survival as a consequence of hyperglycemia (and resultant hyperosmolarity) and metabolic acidosis.

Hyperglycemia

Decreased tissue utilization of glucose and glucose overproduction by the liver characterize the insulin-deficient state. Whereas glucose is released by the liver at a rate of 150–200 mg/min (2 mg/kg/min) in normal postabsorptive subjects, in DKA the rate of glucose production is increased to 400–600 mg/min.[1] Thus hyperglycemia does not

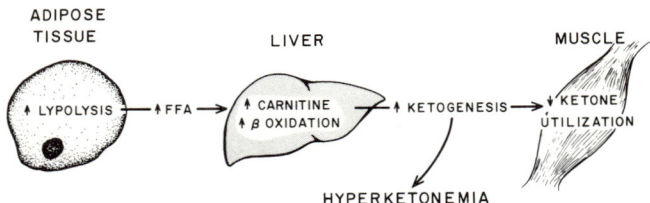

Fig. 12-1. Tissues and processes involved in the development of DKA. Insulin deficiency results in (1) increased lipolysis (adipose tissue), (2) increased β oxidation of fatty acids within mitochondria as a consequence of elevated levels of carnitine (liver), and (3) reduced oxidation of ketones (muscle). The net result is accumulation of ketone acids in blood, resulting in hyperketonemia.

depend on failure to metabolize ingested carbohydrate; it is a result of overproduction of glucose from endogenous precursors. Since protein-derived amino acids are the only precursors available for de novo glucose synthesis, implicit in this increase in gluconeogenesis is dissolution of body protein stores and development of a negative nitrogen balance. A more immediate threat to the patient, however, is the osmotic diuresis that accompanies severe hyperglycemia and leads to urinary losses of water and sodium as well as to development of hyperosmolarity.

Metabolic Acidosis

Coincident with the increase in blood glucose, ketone acids (acetoacetic acid and β-hydroxybutyric acid) progressively accumulate in blood, reaching levels of 8–15 mmoles/liter. The development of hyperketonemia was for many years viewed as a process that was entirely triggered and regulated by the rate of mobilization of fatty acids from adipose tissue. In the last 5 years several studies have indicated that alterations in hepatic metabolism independent of fatty acid delivery are equally important in the regulation of ketogenesis.[2]

It has been suggested that the metabolic site within the liver that is responsible for this activation of ketogenesis resides in the carnitine acyltransferase reaction.[2,3] This enzyme catalyzes the transfer of long-chain fatty acids across the mitochondrial membrane. Since β oxidation of fatty acids occurs solely within the mitochondria, accelerated transfer of free fatty acids across the membrane results in augmented fatty acid oxidation and acetyl coenzyme A (CoA) production. The marked increase in acetyl CoA availability exceeds the capacity for its oxidation to CO_2 via the Krebs cycle, resulting in condensation of acetyl CoA molecules to form ketone acids. The mechanism whereby insulin deficiency leads to augmented activity of the carnitine acyltransferase reaction is believed to involve augmented transfer of carnitine from extrahepatic sites to the liver.[4]

In addition to its being a consequence of increased ketone production, hyperketonemia in diabetes is a consequence of decreased utilization of these organic acids by muscle tissue.[5] Even in patients with mild insulin lack, a diminution in ability to dispose of ketones is demonstrable. This decreased ketone utilization is an even more sensitive index of insulin lack than is ketone overproduction.[5]

The sequence of events leading to the development of hyperketonemia involves three systems: adipose tissue, liver, and muscle (Fig. 12–1). Insulin lack results in augmented lipolysis in adipose tissue, which leads to increased delivery of free fatty acids to the liver. Within the liver an insulin-sensitive increase in carnitine levels results in stimulation of the β oxidative pathway and augmented ketone production. The ketones released by the liver cannot be metabolized at normal rates by muscle tissue, and thus they accumulate within the blood. The end result is a metabolic acidosis in which β-hydroxybutyrate and acetoacetate are the predominant organic acids. It should be noted that these ketone acids are generally present in a ratio of 3:1 favoring β-hydroxybutyrate.

DIAGNOSIS

Prompt diagnosis of DKA requires a high index of suspicion in patients with mental obtundation, dehydration, hyperpnea, vomiting and abdominal pain, or an acetone odor on the breath. The diagnosis is rapidly established by examining three parameters: urinary glucose and ketones, arterial blood pH and blood gases, and serum ketones. The serum ketone level is determined semiquantitatively by adding a drop of serum to a crushed nitroprusside tablet (Acetest) and observing for a strong, moderate, light, or negative reaction for acetone.

The diagnosis of DKA is established if *all* of the following findings are present: 4+ glucose and strong reaction for ketones in urine; pH below 7.3 and P_{CO_2} of 40 mm Hg or less in arterial blood; strongly positive nitroprusside reaction in undiluted serum. These simple measurements permit rapid establishment of a diagnosis before the laboratory reports of blood glucose level and serum bicarbonate determination become available. The need for serial dilutions in performing the Acetest reaction on serum is also eliminated, as repetition of this test is generally unnecessary in observing the patient's response to treatment.

It should be noted that the nitroprusside reaction permits estimation of acetoacetic acid and acetone but does not detect β-hyrodxybutyrate. In situations in which DKA is accompanied by lactic acidosis, a weakly positive reaction may not reflect the magnitude of ketonemia, since the altered redox state favors conversion of acetoacetate to β-hydroxybutrate. On the other hand, an accumulation of ketone acids sufficient to cause metabolic acidosis may be seen in the absence of diabetes in poorly nourished alcoholic patients with repeated bouts of vomiting.[6] In such cases of alcoholic ketoacidosis (in which treatment with insulin is not required), blood glucose levels are below 250 mg/dl, and urine tests do not show a 4+ reaction for glucose.

TREATMENT

Management of DKA consists of administration of insulin to normalize body metabolism, restoration of fluid and electrolyte deficits, a search for a precipitating cause (e.g., occult infection), and avoidance of complications (e.g., cerebral edema, hypoglycemia).[7]

Fluids

Therapy is initiated by rapid infusion of large volumes of hypotonic (0.45 percent) saline solution at rates of 500–1000 ml/hr for the first 2–3 hr. In the patient with hypotension or other evidence of shock (oliguria), normal saline (0.9 percent sodium chloride solution) is the fluid of choice. In the elderly patient or in circumstances of cardiac failure, a central venous catheter should be placed to assess the adequacy of fluid replacement.

Insulin

Treatment with insulin is instituted simultaneously. Intermittent administration of large doses of rapid-acting insulin (50–100 units in adult patients) by the intravenous or subcutaneous route has long been recommended.[7] However, recent studies indicate that continuous intravenous infusion of small amounts of insulin (2–12 units/hr) is a simpler and probably safer approach.[8-10] Since there is some disagreement and controversy regarding the optimal approach to treatment,[11,12] it will be useful to review several aspects of the secretion, action, and turnover of insulin.

INSULIN PHYSIOLOGY

In the normal individual in the postabsorptive state (10–14 hr overnight fast), insulin does not disappear from the circulation but is present in concentrations of 10–20 μunits/ml. These basal levels of insulin are maintained as a consequence of pancreatic secretory rates of approximately 1 unit/hr.[13,14] It is precisely these secretory rates of insulin that in the normal fasting individual serve to restrict glucose production by the liver to 150 mg/min while limiting lipolysis in adipose tissue and ketogenesis in the liver and maintaining ketone utilization in muscle so that total blood ketone acid levels in these circumstances are less than 0.5 mmoles/liter.

With respect to the fed state, insulin levels in blood rise to concentrations of 50–100 μunits/ml, while secretory rates generally increase by no more than fivefold. It is of interest that the effect of insulin on such parameters as glucose uptake and utilization reaches a maximum at high physiologic levels (200–300 μunits/ml). Increments in plasma levels above those concentrations are without further effect.[15]

Concerning the turnover of insulin, it is noteworthy that the half-life of endogenous or exogenous insulin is approximately 3–5 min.[13] Thus after a bolus intravenous injection it can be expected that little residual insulin will be available in plasma after 30 min. Although an effect of insulin (due to distribution in tissue fluid) is likely to persist for an additional 30–45 min,[14] it is unlikely that intravenous bolus injections of insulin will persist in biologic activity for more than 2 hr. It is of interest that bolus injections of insulin in doses of 0.1 units/kg result in initial plasma concentrations in excess of 1500 μunits/ml (well above the physiologic range of insulin action), but they decline rapidly over the ensuing 30 min.

From the above considerations three things are apparent: insulin is a hormone that effectively inhibits ketogenesis when delivered in basal amounts (1 unit/hr). The effect of insulin reaches saturation at high physiologic levels. The turnover of this hormone is extremely rapid, so that the effects of bolus intravenous injections are quickly dissipated.

INSULIN ADMINISTRATION

With respect to the optimal approach to insulin treatment of DKA, the following criteria should be met: (1) certainty of absorption (this is particularly important in a dehydrated, hypovolemic patient); (2) persistence of hyperinsulinemia (rather than hyperinsulinemia followed by hypoinsulinemia); (3) restoration of physiologic insulin levels in blood. On the basis of the considerations discussed above regarding insulin

Table 12-1
Low-Dose Continuous Insulin Infusion Technique

1. Administer loading dose of 6 units of regular insulin intravenously.
2. Add 50 units of regular insulin to 500 ml of saline.
3. Infuse insulin-saline mixture at rate of 60 ml/hr (via pediatric infusion set).
4. Administer non-insulin-containing fluids at rate of 500–1,000 ml/hr.
5. Double insulin infusion rate if blood glucose level fails to decline 30% in 2–4 hr.

secretion, sensitivity, saturation, and turnover, it is apparent that continuous low-dose intravenous administration of insulin fulfills all of these criteria.

The low-dose continuous insulin infusion procedure as initially introduced involved the use of an infusion pump (to ensure delivery rates) and the use of serum albumin (to prevent adsorption of insulin to tubing or glassware).[8-10] Subsequent experience has indicated that simpler procedures in which neither the pump nor the albumin is employed are equally successful.[16,17] The regimen we recommend is as follows: an initial loading dose of 6 units of rapid-acting insulin is given, followed by continuous infusion of rapid-acting insulin (regular insulin or crystalline zinc insulin) in a dose of 6 units/hr. In children a dose of 0.1 unit/kg/hr may be used.[17]

Infusion of these small amounts of insulin is accomplished by adding 50 units of regular insulin to 500 ml of saline solution and infusing the insulin-saline mixture (via a pediatric infusion set) at a rate of 60 ml/hr. The insulin drip is connected in piggyback fashion via a 25-gauge needle directly into the intravenous line, through which fluids are being rapidly administered. In this manner the patient receives the large volume of fluids and electrolytes necessary to restore these deficits, while receiving only small amounts of insulin to correct the metabolic derangements (Table 12-1).

The response to treatment is assessed by monitoring blood glucose, serum electrolytes, arterial pH, and urine glucose and ketones at intervals of 2–4 hr. If the blood glucose level does not decline 30 percent in the first 2–4 hr or 50 percent in 6–8 hr, the insulin infusion rate should be doubled. If hyperglycemia persists, the rate should be doubled at 2-hr intervals. Once the blood glucose level falls to 200 or 300 mg/dl the insulin infusion is discontinued, and infusion of 5 percent dextrose solution is started. Intermittent small doses (10 units) of rapid-acting insulin are administered subcutaneously thereafter, as necessary to control glycosuria. It should be noted that arterial pH and serum bicarbonate level, as well as blood glucose concentration, should be used as indices to determine cessation of insulin infusion. If blood glucose level has fallen to below 300 mg/dl but arterial pH remains below 7.3, then the serum (or plasma) Acetest (nitroprusside) determination should be repeated. If large or moderate amounts of ketones are present (in undiluted serum), then insulin (6 units/hr) together with glucose (200 ml of 5 percent dextrose per hour should be administered. If the nitroprusside reaction is negative or only faintly positive, the findings (euglycemic nonketotic metabolic acidosis) suggest development of an accompanying lactic acidosis requiring treatment with sodium bicarbonate.

CHOICE OF INSULIN REGIMEN

Rapid acceptance of the low-dose insulin procedure in many centers has led to a plea for caution before abandoning conventional treatment with large doses (50–100 units) of insulin administered intermittently by the intravenous and/or subcutaneous routes.[11] Clearly the rate and route of insulin delivery are less important than prompt diagnosis, careful bedside monitoring, and individualization of therapy, regardless of the regimen employed. In the hands of an experienced team, the two insulin regimens (conventional and low-dose) are equally effective.[18] The significance of the findings with the low-dose regimen is not (as has been suggested[11]) to initiate a competition to determine the lowest possible effective insulin dosage; rather, the question posed is the type of regimen likely to be most effective in the widest variety of clinical and hospital settings. This includes consideration of such factors as availability of personnel and techniques for monitoring metabolic parameters, as well as experience in treating such patients.

Continuous low-dose infusion of insulin offers the advantages of simplicity and ease of administration, assurance of absorption, lessened likelihood of hypoglycemia, and physiologic rates of insulin delivery. However, certain precautions must be exercised. Fluids must be administered in volumes of 500–1000 ml/hr (particularly in the first 2–3 hr). In the absence of adequate fluid replacement, patients will not respond to large or small doses of insulin. In addition, the insulin dose should be doubled at 2-hr intervals if the patient fails to improve. Intermittent large doses of insulin should be employed if the patient does not respond to an increase in the infusion rate or if he shows evidence of a worsening clinical status.

Potassium

As a consequence of acidosis, diuresis, and frequent vomiting, body potassium stores are depleted by 5–10 mEq/kg body weight. Nevertheless, the serum potassium concentration is generally normal or elevated because of the shift in potassium from intracellular to extracellular fluid accompanying an increase in hydrogen ion concentration. With correction of acidosis and stimulation of cellular uptake of glucose, serum potassium levels decline. Accordingly, potassium chloride (or phosphate) should be administered 3–4 hr after initiation of therapy (provided the patient is not anuric) at a dose of 40 mEq/liter of intravenous fluid. A total of 120–160 mEq is generally infused in the first 12–18 hr. In the rare patient (<5 percent of cases) in whom hypokalemia is present at the outset, potassium supplements (40 to 60 mEq of potassium chloride per liter) are added to the initial intravenous infusion.

Bicarbonate

Although by definition serum pH is reduced in all patients with DKA, sodium bicarbonate should not be routinely administered. Since acetoacetate and β-hydroxybutyrate are metabolizable anions, restoration of serum bicarbonate concentration toward normal will follow insulin administration in the absence of treatment with alkali-containing solutions. Consequently, infusion of bicarbonate may result in a mild metabolic alkalosis. The shift to the left in the oxygen dissociation curve brought about by alkalinization may limit tissue oxygen delivery, since red cell 2,3-diphosphoglycerate (2,3-DPG) concentration is reduced in DKA and is not immediately restored by insulin treatment.[19] On the other hand, severe reductions in arterial pH may impair myocardial contractility and directly contribute to central nervous system depression. Accordingly, treatment with bicarbonate should be restricted to patients with severe metabolic acidosis, as indicated by an arterial pH of 7.1 or less or a bicarbonate level of less than 5 mEq/liter. In such circumstances 88 mEq of sodium bicarbonate (132 mEq if pH < 7.0) should be added to the initial liter of hypotonic saline. Additional bicarbonate is given only so long as blood pH (measured 2 hr after institution of treatment) remains below 7.25. To avoid the possiblity of aggravating cellular dehydration by infusing a hypertonic solution, it is important to add the bicarbonate to a hypotonic solution of sodium chloride (0.45 percent) rather than infuse it with isotonic (0.9 percent) saline. Since blood lactate levels tend to be slightly elevated in ketonacidotic patients, there is no justification for infusion of sodium lactate in preference to bicarbonate.

REFERENCES

1. Bondy PK, Bloom WL, Whitner VS, et al: Studies on the role of the liver in human carbohydrate metabolism by the venous catheter technic. II. Patients with diabetic ketosis before and after the administration of insulin. J Clin Invest 28:1126–1132, 1949
2. McGarry JD, Foster DW: Regulation of ketogenesis and clinical aspects of the ketotic state. Metabolism 21:471–489, 1972
3. McGarry JD, Foster DW: The metabolism of (-)-octanoylcarnitine in perfused livers from fed and fasted rats. Evidence for a possible regulatory role of carnitine acyltransferase in the control of ketogenesis. J Biol Chem 249:7984, 1977
4. McGarry JD, Robles-Valdes C, Foster DW: Role of carnitine in hepatic ketogenesis. Proc Natl/Acad Sci USA 72:4385, 1975
5. Sherwin RS, Hendler RG, Felig P: Effect of diabetes mellitus and insulin on the turnover and metabolic response to ketones in man. Diabetes (in press)
6. Levy LJ, Duga J, Girgis M, et al: Ketoacidosis associated with alcoholism in nondiabetic subjects. Ann Intern Med 78:213–219, 1973
7. Felig P: Diabetic ketoacidosis. N Engl J Med 290:1360–1363, 1974
8. Page MM, Alberti KG, Greenwood R, et al: Treatment of diabetic coma with continuous low-dose infusion of insulin Br Med J 2:687–690, 1974
9. Kidson W, Casey J, Kraegen E, et al: Treatment of severe diabetes mellitus by insulin infusion. Br Med J 2:691–694, 1974
10. Semple PF, White C, Manderson WG: Continuous intravenous infusion of small doses of insulin in the treatment of diabetic ketoacidosis. Br Med J 2:694–698, 1974
11. Madison LL: Low-dose insulin: A plea for caution. New Engl J Med 294:393–394, 1976
12. Page MM, Pyke DA, Watkins PJ, et al: Treatment of diabetic ketoacidosis. N Engl J Med 294:1183, 1976
13. Sonksen PH, Tompkins CV, Srivatava MC, et al: A comparative study on the metabolism of human insulin and porcine proinsulin in man. Clin Sci Mol Med 45:633–654, 1973
14. Sherwin RS, Kramer KJ, Tobin JD, et al: a model of the kinetics of insulin in man. J Clin Invest 53:1481–1492, 1974
15. Christensen NJ, Orskov H: The relationship between endogenous serum insulin concentration and glucose uptake in the forearm muscles of non-diabetics. J Clin Invest 47:1262–1268, 1968
16. Felig P: Insulin: Rates and routes of delivery N Engl J Med 291:1031–1032, 1974
17. Felig P: Combating diabetic ketoacidosis and other hyperglycemic-ketoacidotic syndromes. Postgrad Med 59:150–153, 1976
18. Soler NG, Fitzgerald MG, Wright AD, et al: Comparative study of different insulin regimens in management of diabetic ketoacidosis. Lancet 2:1221–1224, 1975
19. Alberti KGMM, Darley JH, Emerson PM, et al: 2,3-Diphosphoglycerate and tissue oxygenation in uncontrolled diabetes mellitus. Lancet 2:391–395, 1972

Robert L. Lavine

13
Diabetes and Pregnancy

Prior to the discovery of insulin, pregnancy complicated by diabetes mellitus was a rare occurrence. Fertility in diabetics was greatly diminished; only 1 of 20 diabetic women ever conceived.[1] Those who did could not be considered fortunate, since 1 of 4 died during her pregnancy. Moreover, in those few women who did become pregnant and who survived their pregnancy, the chances of their leaving the hospital with a living infant were less than 50 percent, since the rate of stillbirth or death of the infant during the neonatal period was extremely high.[2]

Fortunately this bleak outlook changed with the discovery of insulin. With the control of diabetes by insulin, problems with fertility vanished, and maternal mortality was reduced to that observed in nondiabetic pregnant women. While there was also some improvement in the extremely high perinatal mortality that obtained in the preinsulin era, an unacceptably high rate of stillbirth and neonatal death still remained. While this problem has been reduced to 10 percent or less in well-equipped centers interested and experienced in the unique problems caused by diabetes complicating pregnancy, perinatal mortality is still significantly greater than that observed in nondiabetic pregnancies. In centers with limited facilities and little experience in handling this problem, the perinatal mortality rate may still be as high as 30 percent.[3]

How the fetus is adversely affected by diabetes is unknown. However, there is no question that an intrauterine environment which has been altered by diabetes is detrimental to the fetus. This is underscored by the observation that fetal complications and perinatal mortality vary inversely with control of the diabetic state.[4] The adverse effect of maternal diabetes on the fetus is also underscored by the observation that, in comparison to pregnancies in normal women, fetal and neonatal losses occur with significantly greater frequency in pregnancies where the maternal diabetes is mild, where diabetes has occurred during the pregnancy (being present neither before conception nor post partum, so-called gestational diabetes), and even where the patient is a prediabetic (i.e., the patient does not have diabetes at the time of pregnancy but develops diabetes at some later date).[5]

METABOLIC CHANGES IN PREGNANCY

In order to understand the changes taking place in pregnant diabetic women, an understanding of the metabolic changes in normal nondiabetic pregnancies is necessary. Pregnancy involves a state of insulin antagonism, i.e., more insulin than normal is required to maintain glucose homeostasis. This insulin antagonistic state is confirmed by the decreased effect of exogenous insulin in lowering blood sugar. As pregnancy progresses, fasting plasma glucose tends to decrease. Associated with fasting is a rapid change to a starvation pattern of carbohydrate metabolism, with increased free fatty acids and ketone levels.[6] This lowered fasting glucose is thought to be due to fetal glucose utilization, in addition to decreased maternal release of alanine, a gluconeogenic precursor.[7] Since the growing fetus needs increasing amounts of maternal glucose, maternal carbohydrate metabolism is shifted toward decreasing maternal peripheral utilization of glucose. In order to keep this process in check and avoid precipitation of diabetes, increasing amounts of insulin must be secreted. Therefore, in pregnancy insulin is secreted in greater than normal amounts in response to glucose, and this heightened secretion increases with the duration of pregnancy, consistent with the increasing insulin antagonistic state.[3] While they are low in the first trimester, there is a tendency for the fasting insulin levels to rise in the second and third trimesters.[8]

In most diabetic pregnancies this compensatory increase in insulin usually does not occur, and diabetes becomes more difficult to control as pregnancy continues. In gestational diabetic pregnancies, however, there is an increase in insulin, but the pattern of release is abnormal and normal glucose tolerance is not maintained. In this group of patients glucose tolerance becomes abnormal and usually deteriorates as pregnancy progresses. Paradoxically, the insulin response to a glucose load is quite large; frequently it is greater than in nondiabetic pregnant women.[3] However, the insulin response resembles that observed in early adult-onset diabetes mellitus, and like that of adult-onset diabetes, it usually shows a somewhat delayed release of insulin. Since rapid release of insulin is important in determining subsequent glucose utilization, this delayed insulin response causes glucose intolerance, despite increased insulin levels. As with adult-onset diabetes, there may also be an insulin overshoot with a subsequent reactive hypoglycemia that may even cause symptoms in gestational diabetic patients. As pregnancy continues, the ability to secrete insulin may diminish in this group; as this point is reached, exogenous insulin becomes necessary.

The major factors responsible for the insulin antagonism of pregnancy are unknown, but several factors have been suggested. Whichever factor or factors are responsible, it is obvious that the insulin antagonism is closely related to placental function. Factors in pregnancy that have been implicated in causing this insulin antagonistic state will be discussed briefly:

1. Estrogen is secreted by the placenta in increasing amounts, causing a slight decrease in glucose tolerance with an increased release of insulin.[9]
2. Progesterone is secreted by the placenta and opposes the glucose-lowering effect of insulin. With progesterone the glucose tolerance usually remains normal, but at the expense of a compensatory increase in insulin release.[10]
3. Human placental lactogen (HPL) is a placental polypeptide secreted into the maternal circulation; it has growth-hormone-like activity as well as luteotropic and mammotropic activity. It is lipolytic and opposes the action of insulin. It also increases

pancreatic glucose-induced insulin release. It is of interest that when HPL was infused into nonpregnant nondiabetic women (normal oral and cortisone glucose tolerance tests), glucose tolerance changed little, but insulin secretion was enhanced to a degree similar to that seen in normal pregnancy. When HPL was infused into latent diabetic women (normal oral glucose tolerance test but abnormal cortisone glucose tolerance test), marked deterioration of glucose tolerance occurred. This was associated with delayed (but increased) secretion of insulin, with curves similar to the curves obtained from gestational diabetics.[11]

4. Free cortisol is slightly increased in pregnancy, and it has insulin antagonistic effects.[12] However, because the increase in the free level of this hormone is small, it probably exerts only a small effect, if any, on the increased insulin antagonism in pregnancy.

Anti-insulin factors that appear to be of little or no significance in the insulin resistance of pregnancy are the following:

1. The placenta has a high capacity to degrade insulin.[16] However, this cannot account for the increased levels of insulin following oral glucose.
2. Growth hormone levels remain normal throughout pregnancy, while responses to insulin hypoglycemia and arginine are suppressed in the third trimester.[13]
3. Glucagon levels increase during pregnancy, but less so than insulin levels.[14]

At any rate, no matter what factors are responsible for the insulin antagonism of pregnancy, more insulin, secreted in a normal fashion, is required to maintain relatively normal carbohydrate homeostasis. If this cannot be accomplished, diabetes ensues.

SCREENING

Perinatal loss of infants even in mild or gestational diabetic pregnancies exceeds that observed in nondiabetic pregnancies, and treatment significantly improves this loss. Therefore it is of paramount importance to identify the diabetic patient. This is no problem in the known diabetic. However, when trying to find those pregnancies complicated by diabetes in patients with no previous history of diabetes, a considerable problem arises. Since only 1 in 200–500 pregnancies is complicated by diabetes,[1] it is obvious that screening every pregnant woman for the presence of diabetes is not justified. However, certain risk factors have been identified that should alert the physician to the possibility of diabetes in a patient and make screening of that patient for diabetes mandatory. The more risk factors present, the greater the likelihood that the patient will have abnormal glucose tolerance or diabetes. These risk factors are listed in Table 13–1. Even though glycosuria is frequently seen during pregnancy because of the lowered renal threshold for glucose, significant glycosuria as defined in Table 13–1 may be associated with abnormal glucose tolerance in up to 21 percent of patients.

In screening patients one must know whether plasma or whole blood is being assayed, since plasma will yield values that average 15–20 percent higher than whole blood glucose values. It must also be remembered that because of the changes in carbohydrate homeostasis in pregnancy the criteria for abnormal glucose tolerance are somewhat different. With this in mind, it is recommended that patients be screened as soon as the question of diabetes arises. Patients should be screened after an overnight fast, using an oral

Table 13–1
Risk Factors for Diabetes Mellitus in Pregnancy*

A. Poor obstetric history (includes history of fetal and/or perinatal loss or toxemia)
B. History of large infant ($\geq$ 9.5 lb)
C. Glycosuria is important if
   1. it appears early in pregnancy
   2. it contains 3+ to 4+ glucose by semiquantitative methods
   3. it is present in second-voided fasting specimen
   4. it is present in two random specimens throughout the day
D. Family history of diabetes mellitus
E. Multiparity
F. Obesity
G. Older age

*Factors A–D are considered the more important risk factors.

glucose tolerance test and 100 g of glucose. An intravenous glucose tolerance test is not recommended, since there are increased numbers of false negative tests as compared to the oral test.[15] This is especially bad, because unrecognized diabetes complicating pregnancy will result in increased perinatal loss. Normal individuals should have *plasma* glucose values at fasting and at 1, 2, and 3 hr after oral glucose no greater than 105, 190, 165, and 145 mg/dl, respectively. If two of these values are exceeded, then the diagnosis of diabetes is made. (Corresponding whole blood glucose values would be 90, 165, 145, and 125 mg/dl at fasting and at 1, 2, and 3 hr post oral glucose).[16] If the glucose tolerance test is equivocal, repeat it. If significant glycosuria develops, if there develop complications of pregnancy that may be associated with diabetes, or if a large-for-date baby is found, also repeat the glucose tolerance test. Two qualifications to these screening recommendations are necessary:

1. If the patient has been carbohydrate-restricted by diet or because of hyperemesis, interpretation of the tolerance test (especially if only mildly abnormal) becomes difficult, since starvation or carbohydrate restriction can decrease insulin reponse to glucose and cause abnormal tolerance. Therefore, perform the test after 3 days of carbohydrate loading.
2. If the patient has symptoms suspicious of diabetes mellitus, she should first be screened with a 2-hr-postprandial glucose determination. If this value exceeds 200 mg/dl (plasma) or 175 mg/dl (whole blood), then diabetes is present. If the 2-hr-postprandial glucose does not exceed these values, then a standard 3-hr glucose tolerance test is necessary. Since the diagnosis of diabetes radically alters the management of the pregnancy, a glucose tolerance test should always be done if the results of the postprandial screen leave any doubt as to the presence or absence of diabetes mellitus.

CLASSIFICATION

While each diabetic pregnancy must be managed on an individual basis, White's classification of the diabetic pregnancy,[17] based on duration of maternal diabetes and the presence or absence of various diabetic vascular complications, is quite helpful. This classification alerts the physician to the fact that in patients with diabetes of longer

Table 13-2
Classification of Diabetic Pregnancies*

Class	Definition
A	Chemical diabetes
B	Diabetes of less than 10 years, with onset at ≥ 20 years of age; no angiopathy
C	Diabetes for 10–19 years, with onset at 10–19 years of age; no angiopathy
D	Diabetes for ≥ 20 years; background retinopathy and calcified peripheral vessels may be present
F	Nephropathy present
R	Malignant retinopathy present

*Adapted from White P: Pregnancy complicating diabetes. Am J Med 7:609–616, 1949.

duration and in those who have angiopathy (as one goes from class A to class R), fetal prognosis is worse, and delivery usually must be performed earlier than in those patients who have diabetes of short duration and no angiopathy. This classification (Table 13–2) is also useful if one is studying diabetes complicating pregnancy.

MANAGEMENT

Successful management of the pregnancy that is complicated by diabetes mellitus involves a coordinated intensive team effort by the internist and the obstetrician with addition of a pediatrician at delivery. Insulin-requiring diabetics should be seen weekly by both obstetrician and internist from the beginning, while patients with diabetes controlled by diet alone should be seen every other week until the 28th week of pregnancy and then weekly. As in the case of nonpregnant diabetics, diet is extremely important. The diet is similar to standard diabetic diets, except that the amount of carbohydrate is increased to 150–200 g to ensure adequate levels of glucose for fetal consumption. The diet should also contain at least 1.5 g of protein per kilogram of body weight. A caloric prescription of 30 cal/kg body weight is advised. Since sodium and fluid retention are a problem in diabetic pregnancies, salt restriction (no added salt, or even more severe restriction) is advised. The object of diet therapy is to aid in the control of blood sugar and to help control weight gain such that no more than 20 pounds are gained during the pregnancy.

In those patients whose glucose levels cannot be normalized by diet, insulin is required. Despite considerable controversy as to the value of normalizing plasma glucose levels in diabetics in general, there is no controversy regarding the benefits of the best possible glucose control in diabetic pregnancies. Therefore insulin is administered in an attempt to control the diabetic state as much as possible; normal fasting and postprandial glucose levels are the goal. Insulin therapy should be carried out with an intermediate-acting insulin (NPH or Lente), while the dosage should be varied frequently to ensure adequate control of blood sugar. It is often necessary to split the insulin dose (two-thirds in the morning and one-third in the evening) or to add regular insulin to the regimen to obtain adequate control. Since the renal threshold for glucose is lowered in pregnancy, blood sugars are monitored more frequently than usual. However, urine sugar and ketone determinations are still important, since 4+ glycosuria associated with acetone means that the diabetes is grossly out of control and needs immediated treatment. On the other hand, if the urine is negative but ketones are present, this means the patient needs a reduction of insulin or an increase in dietary carbohydrate or both. Therefore the patient is advised to check second-voided urine specimens for sugar and acetone before meals and before bed.

Adequate control of diabetes in the manner just described will reduce the chance of complications during pregnancy. However, the incidence of complications is not reduced to normal, and every complication adversely affects the chance for a successful outcome of the pregnancy; therefore, when complications arise, they must be treated intensively, usually in a hospital environment. These complications are listed in Table 13–3. Complications A–D are especially unwanted toward the end of pregnancy, since they adversely affect fetal survival and may force delivery earlier than planned.

Ketoacidosis, especially in the second trimester, is associated with an extremely high incidence of fetal death. In fact, elevated ketones, per se, appear to be detrimental, since elevated ketones correlate directly with the incidence of fetal central nervous system (CNS) malformation in diabetic pregnancies. Hypoglycemia, on the other hand, does not appear to be detrimental to fetal CNS development.[18] Hydramnios is seen in up to 25% of diabetic pregnancies,[19] and if it is present beyond the 32nd week (especially if associated with preeclampsia) it augurs a poor fetal prognosis. Pyelonephritis is especially dangerous to the fetus if it is associated with maternal proteinuria and angiopathy. Dystocia is a frequent problem in pregnancy in women with gestational or short-duration diabetes, since the fetuses of these patients tend to be large. This predisposes to prolonged and difficult labor and birth trauma, both of which adversely affect perinatal survival. Two other factors that are not complications of the diabetic pregnancy but that adversely influence the outcome have been stressed by Pedersen: poor patient cooperation and late presentation for prenatal care.[20]

An extremely important and difficult aspect of management of the pregnant diabetic is the determination of the appropriate time to deliver the patient. This decision is important because of the high incidence of intrauterine fetal death and stillbirth toward the end of the diabetic pregnancy, even in well-controlled cases. The decision is difficult because if one delivers the patient too early in an attempt to avoid intrauterine death, the incidence of neonatal death due mainly to respiratory distress syndrome (RDS) becomes unacceptably high. Therefore the obstetrician has to deliver at the optimum time, when the risks of both intrauterine death and death due to pulmonary immaturity (RDS) are minimal. While this optimal time is thought to be somewhere between the 37th and 38th weeks of pregnancy, the decision of when to deliver still remains quite difficult. This decision is difficult because the dates of the pregnancy are frequently inaccurate. While this is not a significant problem in low-risk normal pregnancies, it poses a serious problem in dating diabetic pregnancies where judgment as to the length of pregnancy is of critical importance. In addition, other signs used by the obstetrician to judge the length of pregnancy may be misleading in diabetic pregnancies. The large size of many fetuses of diabetic women may give a false impression as to the length of gestation. This is true whether the patient be examined at the bedside by the obstetrician or by ultrasound technique. Even checking for centers of ossification in the fetus by x-ray is misleading, because ossification proceeds more rapidly in these fetuses.[4] Finally, maternal complications may force earlier delivery than anticipated, despite the physician's efforts.

In an attempt to make the decision of when to deliver easier, methods to assess fetal well-being have long been sought. Many have been tried, none is ideal, and all have been

Table 13-3
Maternal Complications of Diabetic Pregnancy

Ketoacidosis
Hydramnios
Preeclampsia
Pyelonephritis
Dystocia
Operative delivery (cesarean section)

known to fail when needed most. However, the following are helpful in monitoring fetal well-being:

1. Estriol reflects the functioning of both the fetus and the placenta. Estriol levels increase with the duration of pregnancy. Falling levels indicate distress, while levels less than 5 mg/day (urine) or 2.6 µg/ml (plasma) correlate with imminent fetal death.[21,22] Problems in interpreting estriol levels arise because of the normal variability of estriol concentration. Interpretation requires serial tests, with the objective of looking for a downward trend in levels. The 24-hr urinary estriol determination may be complicated by inaccurate urine collections, by the effects of glucose on the determination (it decreases the level slightly),[21] and by a decrease in levels if renal function is decreased. While plasma estriol is easier to interpret, it must be remembered that the levels will be elevated in the face of decreased renal function. Therefore it is recommended that plasma estriol determinations be obtained at week 28 and weekly from week 32. If complications are present, this test should be repeated more frequently.
2. Human placental lactogen reflects placental function. In nondiabetic pregnancies low or falling levels (<4 mg/ml) have been correlated with fetal distress.[23] A major problem with this test is that in diabetic pregnancies the correlation is not as good unless the patient has long-term diabetes or is hypertensive. Why this is so is unknown.
3. Human chorionic gonadotropin (measured by radioimmunoassay) reflects placental function and may be helpful.[24]
4. Insulin requirements reflect the insulin antagonistic state of pregnancy. After the first trimester, requirements for insulin increase dramatically in most patients. Falling requirements late in pregnancy are frequently associated with placental dysfunction.
5. The oxytocin challenge test with fetal monitoring reflects the well-being of the fetus, as well as the ability of the fetus to withstand vaginal delivery.[4] Fetal distress during this test is indicated by deceleration of fetal heart rate during uterine contraction.

Other tests have been devised to assess fetal maturity. These tests require amniocentesis. An extremely important procedure for determining fetal pulmonary maturity, which correlates inversely with the incidence of RDS in the neonatal period, is determination of lecithin/sphingomyelin ratio (L/S ratio).[25] The L/S ratio increases as the fetal lung produces surfactant. When the L/S ratio is ≥ 2.0, the chances of RDS developing after delivery are small. Therefore if the L/S ratio is ≥ 2.0 there should be little hesitancy in delivering the baby; if it is less, this is an indication that RDS is likely, and the pregnancy should probably be carried further unless maternal complications or placental insufficiency make prolongation hazardous for fetal survival.

DELIVERY

Ideally, the patient should be admitted to the hospital as early as possible prior to expected delivery for optimum metabolic control and assessment of fetal status. Certain European centers recommend admission at 32 weeks.[4] Since this is usually not feasible in this country, it is recommended that the patient be admitted at least 1 week prior to expected delivery. If complications are present, she should be admitted earlier. During this time control of diabetes is optimized, the fetal status is evaluated, and the mode of delivery is decided. While the mode of delivery is an obstetric decision, vaginal delivery is not contraindicated in the diabetic pregnancy and should be the mode of delivery whenever feasible. If the patient is to be delivered by cesarean section, the section should be scheduled for the morning in order to make diabetic control easier. Since separation of the placenta causes the insulin antagonism to be rapidly terminated, the patient's postpartum insulin requirements will be much less. In fact, for the first 5–7 days post partum, requirements will usually be less than prepregnancy insulin requirements. Therefore insulin should be withheld prior to the section, and one-half to two-thirds of the prepregnancy insulin dose should be administered immediately after delivery in the recovery room. The patient should receive intravenous dextrose in an amount of 150 g/day, and supplemental regular insulin may be given as necessary to control blood sugar (not usually necessary). When the patient is ready to eat, she is prescribed a nonpregnancy diabetic diet with a total caloric content adequate to maintain ideal body weight. This diet will have a decreased carbohydrate content as compared to her pregnancy diet (about 50% of total calories are supplied by carbohydrate in standard diabetic diets).

If the patient is in active labor she should be given one-half to two-thirds of her prepregnancy dose of insulin and covered with glucose infusion as recommended above. If labor is being induced, however, the recommendation for the insulin dose is somewhat more difficult, since labor and delivery may not occur. Therefore it is suggested that one-half to two-thirds of the patient's pregnancy dose be administered, unless the obstetrician is quite sure that she will deliver. Again, following plasma glucose levels closely and administering supplements of regular insulin, if necessary, are mandatory. If the physician has not been able to prepare the patient with the appropriate dose of insulin and she had received her full dose of insulin (e.g., in an emergency delivery), then in the postpartum period she must be observed closely for possible development of hypoglycemia.

Within 5–7 days after delivery insulin requirements usually return to their prepregnancy levels. Lactation and nursing may lower insulin requirements, but usually not significantly. However, lactation, with its associated lactosuria, will give 4+ reactions by Clinitest or Benedict's reagent; so the patient must be advised not to increase her insulin because of 4+ urines. She should also be advised to obtain frequent blood sugars during this period so that her diabetes can be properly controlled.

MANAGEMENT OF THE NEWBORN

Since infants born to diabetic mothers have special problems, a pediatrician should be present at the delivery, and the infant should be cared for in a special-care nursery. Table 13–4 lists problems frequently encountered in infants of diabetic mothers in the neonatal period. After a rocky neonatal period, however, these infants do as well as

Table 13-4
Complications Observed More Frequently in Infants of Diabetic Mothers

Neonatal hypoglycemia
Respiratory distress syndrome
Excessive size—mothers usually have had short-duration diabetes
Birth trauma
Birth defects—twice as frequent as compared to infant of nondiabetic mother
Neonatal hyperbilirubinemia
Neonatal hypocalcemia and tetany
Acidosis

infants of nondiabetic mothers. As a group, they progress in a manner similar to the offspring of nondiabetic mothers and have the same or only a slightly greater chance of developing diabetes mellitus at a later date, unless the father is also a diabetic.

EFFECT OF PREGNANCY ON MATERNAL DIABETES

While pregnancy may precipitate diabetes or worsen diabetic control, the anti-insulin effects of pregnancy are reversed rapidly after placental separation, usually leaving no lasting ill-effect on the patient. In the gestational diabetic, glucose tolerance reverts to normal within 1–2 months post partum (in fact, gestational diabetes is diagnosed in this manner). In diabetic patients pregnancy usually does not cause any permanent deterioration of the patient's health, except in those with retinopathy. In diabetes with nephropathy, renal function will deteriorate during pregnancy, and azotemia may force early delivery. However, after delivery, renal function returns to its prepregnancy level.[26] In patients with preexisting retinopathy the retinopathy may progress, and if it is malignant it could lead to blindness.[26] This requires close observation, and therapeutic abortion may be necessary if malignant retinopathy progresses rapidly.

SUMMARY

From the preceding discussion of the problem of diabetes complicating pregnancy, it is obvious that the metabolic abnormalities caused by diabetes mellitus greatly complicate the usual course and management of pregnancy. It is also obvious that the diabetic state in pregnancy adversely affects and correlates inversely with fetal and neonatal survival. Increased understanding of the metabolic changes in pregnancy, improvement in the medical and obstetric care of the pregnant diabetic patient, and improvement in the pediatric care of her infant have markedly improved the bleak outlook of the diabetic pregnancy. Even so, this intensive team effort has not yet reduced this loss to that seen in nondiabetic pregnancies. With increasing knowledge concerning fetal monitoring, better assessment of placental function and fetal maturity, and improved methods of treating diabetes, it should be possible to reduce this fetal and neonatal loss to that observed in normal nondiabetic pregnancies.

REFERENCES

1. Gellis SS, Hsia DY: The infant of the diabetic mother. J Dis Child 97:1–41, 1952
2. Joslin EP: The treatment of diabetes mellitus (ed 3). Philadelphia, Lea & Febiger, 1923, p 784
3. Carrington ER: Diabetes in pregnancy. Clin Obstet Gynecol 16:28–46, 1973
4. Brudenell M, Beard R: Diabetes in pregnancy. Clin Endocrinol Metab 1:673–695, 1972
5. Horger ED, Kellett WW, Williamson HO: Diabetes in pregnancy. Obstet Gynecol 30:46–53, 1967
6. Freinkel N, Herrera E, Knopp RH, Ruder HJ: Metabolic realignment in pregnancy: A clue to diabetogenesis, in Camerini-Davalos RA, Cole HS (eds): Advances in Diabetes, Supplement I. Early Diabetes. New York, Academic, 1970, p 335
7. Felig P, Kim YJ, Lynch V: Amino acid metabolism during starvation in human pregnancy. J Clin Invest 51:1195–1202, 1972
8. Tsai A, Reuler J, Rubenstein A: Diabetes and pregnancy. J Reprod Med 11:23–28, 1973
9. Buchler D, Warren JC: Effects of estrogen on glucose tolerance. Am J Obstet Gynecol 95:479–483, 1966
10. Kalkhoff RK, Jacobson M, Lemper D: Relative effects of progesterone, pregnancy and the augmented insulin response. J Clin Endocrinol Metab 31:24–28, 1970
11. Kalkhoff RK, Richardson BL, Beck P: Relative effects of pregnancy, HPL and prednisolone on CHO tolerance in normal and subclinical diabetic subjects. Diabetes 18:153–163, 1969
12. O'Connell M, Welsh GW: Unbound plasma cortisol in pregnant and Enovid E treated women as determined by ultrafiltration. J. Clin Endocrinol Metab 29:563–568, 1969
13. Yen SCC, Samaan N, Pearson OH: Growth hormone levels in pregnancy. J Clin Endocrinol Metab 27:1341–1347, 1967
14. Kuhl L, Holst JJ: Plasma glucagon and the insulin:glucagon ratio in gestational diabetes. Diabetes 25:16–23, 1976
15. Benjamin F, Casper DJ: Comparative validity of oral and intravenous glucose tolerance tests in pregnancy. Am J Obstet Gynecol 97:448–492, 1967
16. Wilkerson HLC, O'Sullivan JB: A study of glucose tolerance and screening criteria in 752 unselected pregnancies. Diabetes 12:213–219, 1963
17. White P: Pregnancy complicating diabetes. Am J Med 7:609–616, 1949
18. Churchill JA, Berendes HW, Nemore J: Neurophysiological deficits in children of diabetic mothers. A report from the Collaborative Study for Cerebral Palsy. Am J Obstet Gynecol 105:257–268, 1969
19. Crenshaw C, Parker RT, Carter B: Diabetes mellitus and pregnancy. Obstet Gynecol 20:334–341, 1962
20. Pedersen J: Fetal mortality in diabetic pregnancies. Diabetes 3:199–204, 1954
21. Greene JW, Jr. and Touchstone JC: Urinary estriol as an index of placental function. Amer J Obstet Gynec 85:1–9, 1963
22. Nachtigall L, Bassett M, Hogsander U, et al: Plasma estriol levels in normal and abnormal pregnancies. An index of fetal welfare. Amer J Obstet Gynec 101:638–648, 1968
23. Persson B, Lunell NO, Aubert ML, et al: Determination of plasma human chorionic somatomammotrophin and urinary estriol in diabetic pregnancies. Acta Obstet Gynecol Scand 52:63–67, 1973
24. Kahn CB, White P, Younger M: Laboratory assessment of diabetic pregnancy: A brief review. Diabetes 21:31–38, 1972
25. Gluck L, Kulovich MV, Borer RC Jr, et al: Diagnosis of the respiratory distress syndrome by amniocentesis. Am J Obstet Gynecol 109:440–445, 1971
26. White P: Pregnancy and diabetes. Medical aspects. Med Clin North Am 49:1015–1024, 1965

Frank L. Myers

14
Current Treatment of Diabetic Retinopathy

This chapter will concern some aspects of the current treatment of diabetic retinopathy, beginning with a brief discussion of its incidence, pathogenesis, and natural history.

It is perhaps somewhat of a cliché to tell practicing internists that the late vascular complications of diabetes are presenting an increasing challenge in the management of these patients. However, it is only in the last 5 years or so that ophthalmologists generally have become aware of the increasing magnitude of the problem. When the 1970 Model Reporting Area statistics on the causes of blindness were made available,[1] the importance of diabetic retinopathy as a cause of blindness became obvious, and a surge of interest in the condition began. These figures showed that of the four most common causes of new additions to the blindness registers in 1970 diabetic retinopathy ranked second. Of those additions in the 20- to 64-year age group, diabetes was the leading cause of new cases of blindness, and in those patients with marked decrease in vision (5/200 or less), diabetes was again the leading cause. As a group, diabetics run a risk of becoming blind that is 10 times greater than the risk in the general population.[2] The incidence of retinopathy in the diabetic population has been variously estimated, but in a study by White[3] of 478 juvenile-onset diabetics who survived 30 years or more approximately 10 percent had no retinopathy, 60 percent had nonproliferative retinopathy, and 30 percent had proliferative retinopathy. Twenty-five percent of those with proliferative retinopathy were blind, and 10 percent of the total were blind. Thus diabetic retinopathy has become a major cause for concern and the subject of considerable study.

It is now a well-known fact that (at least in juvenile-onset diabetics) the presence of retinopathy and probably to some extent the severity of retinopathy are related to the duration of the diabetes. While 10–15 years duration before retinopathy appears is the figure usually given, a study[4] at our institution of 191 juvenile-onset insulin-dependent diabetics showed that with careful ophthalmoscopy and fundus photography 70 percent had evidence of retinopathy by 5–7 years and 20 percent had evidence of proliferative retinopathy after 15 years or more of diabetes. Therefore, while referral for ophthalmologic examination is usually not necessary in the early years of diabetes, all diabetics

---

Supported in part by grant 5-P15-EY-00342 from the National Eye Institute.

should probably be referred after 10–15 years duration and should be seen at 1–5-year intervals after that, depending on the findings.

The pathogenesis of the microangiopathy in the diabetic retina consists primarily of capillary closure, but the cause remains obscure. Although diabetes is an inherited disease, animals made diabetic will eventually develop retinopathy, thus implicating the metabolic abnormality as the major causative factor. Engerman[5] has shown that in dogs made diabetic by alloxan the development of retinopathy appears to be inhibited by maintenance of good control of the diabetes. This, of course, may have certain clinical implications.

The natural history of diabetic retinopathy has been fairly well worked out, although some of the details of the incidence and progression of the many manifestations of the disease are not yet clear. Retinopathy usually begins with what are termed nonproliferative changes, consisting of microaneurysms, small intraretinal hemorrhages, hard exudates (edema residue deposits), and soft exudates (microinfarcts). As capillary endothelial cell damage develops, plasma constituents leak out of the vascular system into the retina, resulting in retinal edema. If this encroaches on the macula, central visual acuity is blurred, and eventually degenerative changes occur, permanently impairing vision. This accounts for more than one-fifth of cases of visual loss in diabetics.[6]

Some patients with nonproliferative changes (perhaps as high as one-third) go on to develop proliferative retinopathy. This is characterized by growth of new-formed vessels on the surface of the retina. These are accompanied by fibrous tissue, and as time passes the vessels may regress to a greater or lesser degree and the fibrous tissue component may increase. These changes by themselves do not cause visual problems, but in many cases the vitreous jell for some reason begins to shrink, pulling the new vessels and fibrous tissue forward away from the surface of the retina. If this pull is strong enough, it may tear a vessel, resulting in a vitreous hemorrhage. After a time the pull may be transmitted through the new vessels and fibrous tissue to the retina, detaching the retina and further impairing vision. This process usually proceeds in fits and starts and may stop at any point along the line, thus making the manifestations of the disease extremely variable. Eventually many eyes will reach a sclerotic "burned-out" phase in which the retina may look very ischemic and there may be variable degrees of fibrous tissue and retinal detachment. Vision may vary from moderate loss to no light perception.

Before discussing the current treatment of diabetic retinopathy, I would like to say a word about prevention. Considerable controversy exists concerning the role of control in the prevention of retinopathy. Few solid data have been brought forth to support the idea that control ultimately makes a difference. A controlled trial has never been done, and it would be very difficult to design and execute. Retrospective studies and anecdotal data support the notion that strict control is worthwhile. As mentioned previously, studies in experimental diabetic retinopathy in dogs also tend to support this idea. Engerman kept a colony of alloxan-induced diabetic dogs for 5 years and found a definite statistical decrease in the number of aneurysms, acellular capillaries, and ghost pericytes in animals kept meticulously controlled, as compared to those kept poorly controlled. Thus good control appeared to have an inhibitory effect on development of the early stages of retinopathy. This is only suggestive as far as humans are concerned, but it is an area needing considerable further work. In the meantime we tend to encourage the maintenance of good control in our patients.

The management of visual loss in diabetes involves treatment of the following conditions: (1) macular edema; (2) neovascularization of the retina, which may lead to vitreous hemorrhage; (3) vitreous hemorrhage; (4) retinal detachment; (5) neovascular glaucoma. The latter is often an end-stage condition resulting from new vessel growth on the iris (rubeosis iridis), and until recently it was considered virtually incurable. Standard treatment aims at controlling intraocular pressure medically with topical steroids, atropine, and oral carbonic anhydrase inhibitors. In spite of the legitimate concern about the use of carbonic anhydrase inhibitors in these patients, we have prescribed them for long periods of time without difficulties. Surgical treatment is a last-ditch effort at best, but recent reports of successful photocoagulation treatment in the early stages of this condition are encouraging.

Macular edema occurs most commonly in obese adult-onset diabetics with nonproliferative retinopathy. Areas of retinal edema surrounding leaky microaneurysms form in the posterior retina. Hard exudate edema residue deposits coalesce at the perimeter of these areas, and if the edema or the exudates encroach on the macula, loss of central visual acuity results. Microaneurysms may form in clumps, causing rings of hard exudate to develop, or the microaneurysms may be scattered, resulting in diffuse edema and exudates. Medical treatment with improvement in diabetic control may be beneficial in some cases. In some cases the fact that vision begins to deteriorate is the only thing that will motivate the patient to take dietary control and weight management seriously. Dietary reduction in cholesterol and triglycerides and/or use of clofibrate may result in a reduction in hard exudate deposits in the retina. However, this does not influence retinal edema, and it is questionable if any long-term benefit to visual acuity occurs from a reduction in hard exudates. Diuretics can be tried if the patient is not already taking them for blood pressure control, but they rarely have any effect. Occasionally they have a temporary effect in the diffuse macular edema seen in younger juvenile-onset patients.

Photocoagulation treatment to obliterate leaky microaneurysms seems to have the best chance of restoring or stabilizing visual acuity in diabetic macular edema, particularly if clumps of microaneurysms with surrounding macular edema and rings of hard exudate encroaching on the macula are present, and treatment is directed at these. Xenon arc or argon laser photocoagulation can be used. When scattered microaneurysms and diffuse edema are present, the prognosis is not good, and argon laser photocoagulation is recommended because its beam can be focused into a pencil of light small enough that individual microaneurysms can be treated. Unfortunately, with intravenous fluorescein angiography many of these cases show large areas of retinal capillary nonperfusion, indicating considerable ischemia. Photocoagulation in this instance generally does not eliminate the edema. Studies by Patz et al.,[7] Rubenstein and Myska,[8] and Cheng et al.[9] indicate that photocoagulation is probably worthwhile in cases with only mild or moderate initial vision losses and without large areas of ischemic retina.

Even though many patients with macular edema are disappointed by the results of this treatment, at least they do not go completely blind unless neovascular glaucoma intervenes. On the other hand, those patients afflicted with proliferative retinopathy are faced with this reality because of vitreous hemorrhage or retinal detachment. Medical treatments involving blood vessel strengtheners (such as vitamin C and bioflavinoids, anticoagulants, enzymes, thyroid, vitamin B_{12}, vitamin E, etc.) are virtually worthless, and improvement of diabetic control probably has no effect once proliferative changes are established. Bed rest with head elevation and bilateral patching in the first 24–48 hr after an initial vitreous hemorrhage is of use in hastening the settling-out of the hemorrhage to allow more rapid identification of the bleeding source. Longer periods of inactivity are not warranted because of the attendant general complications and disruption of diabetic management. Several years ago pituitary ablation was advocated in the treatment of certain moderately advanced cases. Studies by Kohner et al.[10] indicated a likely beneficial effect, although the mechanism is not known. However, there has been a marked waning of enthusiasm for pituitary ablation in the past 4–5 years because of the considerable morbidity and not infrequent mortality associated with the procedure. Instead, photocoagulation treatment (especially panretinal photocoagulation) has come to be used with increasing frequency in cases in which vitreous hemorrhage does not cloud the ocular media to any great extent.

Until early in 1976 it was not known conclusively that photocoagulation treatment was beneficial. However, the initial results of a nationwide randomized clinical trail of photocoagulation in proliferative diabetic retinopathy that was initiated 5 years earlier, the Diabetic Retinopathy Study (DRS), have recently become available.[11] These results indicate that in the more than 1700 patients recruited for the study, treatment with either xenon arc photocoagulation or argon laser photocoagulation resulted in an overall 61 percent reduction in blindness in treated eyes as compared to untreated eyes over a 2-year follow-up period. In certain well-defined types of proliferative retinopathy, treatment afforded as much as 70% reduction in the occurrence of blindness (defined as visual acuity less than 5/200 at two or more consecutive 4-month follow-up visits). Side effects such as mild to moderate losses of visual acuity and loss of peripheral field vision did occur in the treated group. The study is continuing, and further results can be expected.

Once severe vitreous hemorrhage or retinal detachment develops in the diabetic eye from retinopathy, photocoagulation treatment cannot be utilized. Until a few years ago no treatment was available for these desperate cases, but now a new surgical procedure called vitrectomy is being utilized with increasing frequency throughout the country. In this operation a surgical instrument, of which there are several designs available, is inserted into the eye (Fig. 14–1). Opaque vitreous jell and old blood are nibbled and sucked out and replaced with clear physiologic solution. Fibrous adhesions between the vitrious and retina that are pulling on and detaching the retina can often be cut.

In some instances of diabetic retinal detachment with tractional hole formation, conventional scleral buckling operations can result in reattachment. Many cases cannot be successfully reattached, and vitrectomy may offer hope for these eyes.

Sometimes dramatic improvement in vision can occur in patients who have been blind from hemorrhage for 3–4 years. The overall improvement rate with this type of surgery done for long-term vitreous hemorrhage is close to 70%.[12] However, the yield of patients who get return of vision to 20/40 or better is small, and the optimum time and specific indications for doing this operation remain unclear. In order to try to determine whether early vitrectomy can held prevent the development of late complications and result in better visual salvage, another large-scale cooperative clinical trial called the Diabetic Retinopathy Vitrectomy Study (DRVS) has been organized by the National Eye Institute. Recruitment began in November 1976.

The treatment of diabetic retinopathy is often disappointing because the underlying disease process is a microangiopathy resulting in capillary closure and increasing ocular and retinal ischemia. Thus, even though we may eliminate edema, destroy new vessels and prevent hemorrhage, and reattach the retina, there may not be marked improvement in vision. Because of the chronicity and variability of the condition, any form of treatment, whether medical or surgical, must be subjected to a randomized controlled study before any conclusions can be drawn concerning efficacy. Diabetic retinopathy remains a challenge to those of us fighting the complications of this disease. But ours is a rear-guard

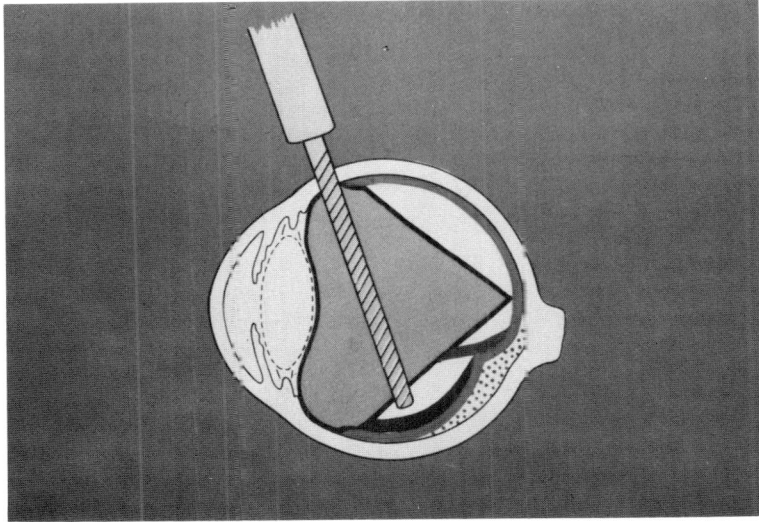

Fig. 14-1. Insertion of surgical instrument in vitrectomy.

action, and the ultimate cure or prevention will probably be predicated on a more basic understanding of the underlying disease process. For this we must once again turn to the basic scientist for help.

REFERENCES

1. Kahn HA, Moorhead HB: Statistics on blindness in the Model Reporting Area, 1969-1970. USDHEW publication (NIH) 73-427. Washington DC, US Government Printing Office, 1973
2. Cairo FI, Pirie A, Ramsell TG: Diabetes and the eye. Blackwell Scientific, Oxford, 1969, p 3
3. White P: Natural course and prognosis of juvenile diabetes. Diabetes 5:445, 1956
4. Davis MD, MacCormick AJ, Harris WAC, et al: Prevalence of diabetic retinopathy in 191 insulin dependent patients. (unpublished data)
5. Engerman RL: Animal models of diabetic retinopathy. Trans Am Acad Ophthalmol Otolaryngol 81:710, 1976
6. Myers FL, Davis, MD, Magli YL: The natural course of diabetic retinopathy: A clinical study of 321 eyes followed one year or more, in Goldberg M, Fine SL (eds): Symposium on the Treatment of Diabetic Retinopathy. USPHS publication 1890. Washington DC, US Government Printing Office, 1969
7. Patz A, Schatz H, Berkow J, et al: Macular edema—an overlooked complication of diabetic retinopathy. Trans Am Acad Ophthalmol Otolaryngol 77:34, 1973
8. Rubenstein K, Myska V: Prognosis and treatment of diabetic maculopathy. Br J Ophthalmol 58:76, 1974
9. Cheng H, Kohner EM, Keen H, et al: Photocoagulation in treatment of diabetic maculopathy. Interim report of a multicentre controlled study. Lancet 2:1110, 1975
10. Kohner EM, Joplin GF, Black RK, et al: Pituitary ablation in the treatment of diabetic retinopathy. A randomized trial. Trans Ophthalmol Soc UK 92:79, 1972
11. Diabetic Retinopathy Study Research Group: Preliminary report on effects of photocoagulation therapy. Am J Ophthalmol 81:383, 1976
12. Myers FL, Bresnick GH: Vitrectomy in diabetic retinopathy. Trans Am Acad Ophthalmol Otolaryngol 81:OP-399, 1976

Peter N. Herbert

15
Hyperlipoproteinemia: A Return to the Basics

Hyperlipidemia derives its enormous clinical relevance from one source: it is causally related to the development of coronary heart disease. Arguments questioning and denying this relationship surface constantly, but they can be distilled to an absurd application of Koch's postulates and a blind denial of an overwhelming amount of experimental and epidemiologic data.[1-7] Certainly other factors, including hypertension, diabetes mellitus, and cigarette smoking, are critical to the observed morbidity and mortality, but the indispensable reagent in the atherosclerotic reaction is the cholesterol carried in the serum lipoproteins.[8-10] And while it is yet to be proved in man that lowering blood lipids will delay or abate the development of ischemic heart disease, there is no ethical justification for denying aggressive management to the countless numbers of individuals who are at apparent high risk.

Virtually all forms of hyperlipidemia, genetic or acquired, can be approached without recourse to specialized diagnostic testing or intricate therapeutic protocols. This requires only the mental translation of plasma lipids to lipoproteins and a knowledge of the few dietary maneuvers and drugs that can alter lipoprotein synthesis or catabolism. This chapter is designed to present the clinically relevant properties of the plasma lipids and lipoproteins, together with a practical approach to the management of hyperlipidemia. A cursory review of the current medical literature reveals that the subject of hyperlipidemia has characteristically been laden with fashionable hypotheses, heresies, claims and counterclaims, and horrible new uncertainties. The apparent confusion beclouds the ease with which hyperlipidemia is diagnosed and the fact that the available therapeutic modalities can normalize plasma lipid levels in the vast majority of hyperlipidemics.

LIPIDS

Fatty Acids

The importance of fatty acids to the body economy is related to their high caloric value, and when generously released from adipose tissue depots in the fasting state they can supply 50–90% of the body's energy requirements. They are potent stimulants of hepatic triglyceride and very low density lipoprotein (VLDL) synthesis. When their release from adipose tissue is pathologically augmented in such diverse settings as insulinopenic diabetes mellitus, hyperthyroidism, and states characterized by high circulating catecholamines, they may produce or aggravate plasma hypertriglyceridemia. In most circumstances, however, fatty acids are quietly shuttled to and from adipose tissue neatly complexed to albumin; they turnover very rapidly in plasma and contribute little to the plasma total lipid content. Laboratory measurement of plasma free fatty acids is rarely, if ever, clinically relevant. Teleologically it is most perplexing why fatty acids need ever be transported in plasma esterified to glycerol as triglyceride. In that rare lipoprotein deficiency state abetalipoproteinemia, plasma triglyceride concentrations are vanishingly low, but there is no consequent disruption of the transport and storage of simple fat.

Triglyceride

In nature the bulk of fatty acids is found esterified to glycerol, predominantly as triglyceride (Fig. 15-1). In contrast to the situation for transport of fatty acids, which is readily accomplished without esterification, esterification is necessary for efficient cellular storage of large quantities of fatty acids. Esterification, producing the "neutral" and "apolar" triglyceride, permits the cell to accommodate large quantities of fat with no increased need for ions to neutralize charge or for water to provide hydration (as is necessary, for example, when glycogen is stored).

Triglyceride, or simple fat, provides 35–50% of the calories in the average American's diet. There is little caloric difference between triglycerides of diverse origin. Dietary triglycerides, however, can profoundly affect the metabolism of the cholesterol-rich plasma lipoproteins, and a nodding familiarity with their sources and properties is germane to a rational approach to the hyperlipidemias.

The fatty acids esterified to the glycerol backbone determine the physical and biochemical properties of the triglyceride. Clinically, fatty acids have been conveniently grouped into the broad categories of saturated, monounsaturated, and polyunsaturated (Fig. 15-1). depending on their degree of hydrogenation. Saturated fats have high melting points, are generally solid at room temperature, and in the diet are derived almost exclusively from the meat and milk of animals. The two notable vegetable fats containing large quantities of saturated fat are coconut oil and cocoa butter. The major saturated fatty acid in animal milk and meat is palmitic (C: 16) acid, and innumerable studies have demonstrated the capacity of saturated fats to elevate serum cholesterol.[12-15]

It is not widely appreciated that oleic acid (Fig. 15-1), which is monounsaturated, accounts for approximately 50% of the fat in meats, irrespective of species origin, and accounts for a highly variable fraction (5–90%) of the fatty acids in "vegetable oils." Recognition of this fact is important, since the effect of monounsaturated fats on the plasma cholesterol level appears to be minimal.[12,13]

Polyunsaturated triglycerides, in general, are of vegetable origin, have low melting points (Fig. 15-1), and are liquid at room temperature. There is considerable variation in the polyunsaturated fat (principally linoleic acid, Fig. 15-1) content of vegetable oils, and since polyunsaturated fats have a hypocholesterolemic effect, this information will be discussed in greater detail when the treatment of hypercholesterolemia is considered.

Hyperlipoproteinemia: A Return to the Basics

FATTY ACIDS

Type	Name	Structure	Melting Point °C
Saturated	Stearic	$CH_3-(CH_2)_{16}-COOH$	70
Mono-unsaturated	Oleic	$CH_3-(CH_2)_7-CH=CH-(CH_2)_7-COOH$	14
Poly-unsaturated	Linoleic	$CH_3-(CH_2)_4-CH=CH-CH_2-CH=CH-(CH_2)_7-COOH$	−5

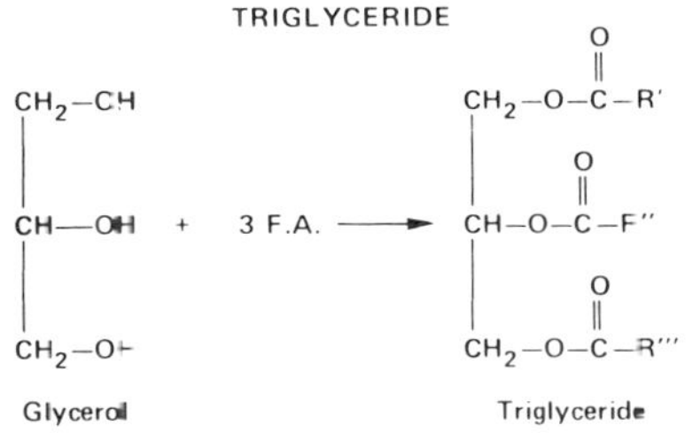

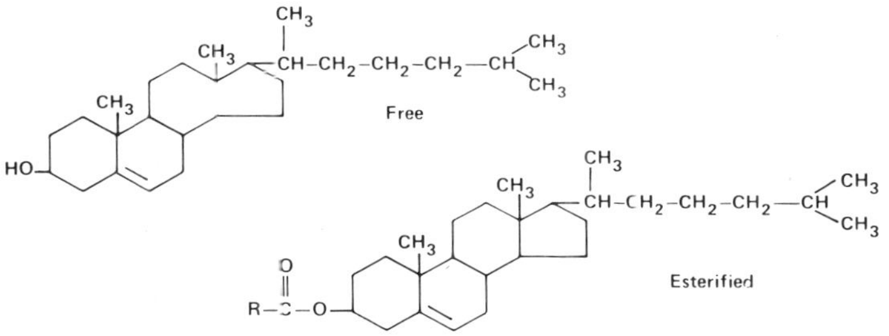

Fig. 15–1. Clinically important plasma lipids. Fatty acid melting points from Fasman.[14]

Cholesterol

Cholesterol, the chemical culprit in the atherosclerosis scenario, is a structural component of most animal cell membranes; in nature it occurs almost exclusively in products of animal origin. Apparently all mammalian tissues are capable of de novo cholesterol biosynthesis; a deficiency state has never been described, and cholesterol is the chemical precursor for synthesis of adrenal and gonadal steroids, bile acids, and a variety of other substances requiring the sterol nucleus (Fig. 15–1). New cholesterol synthesis in the adult animal takes place almost solely in the liver and intestine.[16] Since the cholesterol sterol nucleus is not significantly degraded by mammals, it can be removed from the body only by hepatic excretion through the bile and into the intestine. Most of the pivotal questions relating to plasma cholesterol remain unanswered. Why is tissue cholesterol (with few exceptions) free, while 75% of that in plasma is esterified? Is the cholesterol in plasma actually being transported? If so, between what sites? Does the cholesterol of plasma have an important structural role in lipoproteins comparable to that in tissue plasma membranes? What factors control the plasma cholesterol concentration, and what prompts plasma cholesterol removal and excretion by the liver?

Table 15-1
Plasma Lipoproteins

	Chylomicrons	Very Low Density Lipoproteins	Low-Density Lipoproteins	High-Density Lipoproteins
Characteristics	Scatter light (i.e., produce turbidity); aggregate at 4°C and "cream out" on top of plasma; remain at origin in most electrophoretic systems	Scatter light and produce turbidity; do *not* "cream out" in the cold; pre-β or α-2 mobility on electrophoresis	Do *not* scatter light or produce turbidity, even at very high concentrations; "β" mobility on electrophoresis	Do not scatter light; α-1 mobility on electrophoresis
Tissue origin	From the small intestine *during* absorption of dietary fat	Most from liver; small quantities from intestine	See VLDL; not synthesized per se by any organ or tissue	Synthesized by both liver and intestine
Function	Transport of dietary fat	Transport of fat (i.e., excess calories) from liver to periphery	Uncertain; *garbage* (remnant) from VLDL catabolism	Uncertain; probably modulate chylomicron and VLDL metabolism
Fate	Half-life of 15–30 min; muscle and adipose tissue clear the triglyceride; liver clears the remnants	Half-life of 1–4 hr; triglyceride cleared by same tissues catabolizing chylomicrons	Half-life of 3–4 days; catabolized by peripheral tissues and liver	Half-life of ~ 4 days; degraded by liver and peripheral tissues

Table 15-2
Lipoprotein Composition*

	Chylomicrons	VLDL	LDL	HDL
Cholesterol	5	15	48	20
Triglyceride	86	59	7	3
Phospholipid	7	15	23	27
Protein	2	10	22	50

*Percentage of dry weight.

PLASMA LIPOPROTEINS

Cholesterol and triglyceride cannot be transported in plasma in free form because they are lipids and hence are insoluble in aqueous solutions. Detergents are necessary to promote their miscibility, and the important biologic detergents are the phospholipids and specific proteins. The resultant complexes of free and esterified cholesterol, triglyceride, phospholipid, and protein are the plasma lipoproteins. The lipoproteins are frequently and inappropriately termed molecules, for the constituent biochemicals are not held together by covalent bonds, but rather by complex electrostatic and hydrophobic interactions.

Chylomicrons and VLDL

While they are secreted from different tissues (Table 15-1), chylomicrons and VLDL share many chemical and physiologic features. Triglyceride accounts for 60-80 percent of their mass (Table 15-2), and hypertriglyceridemia can be equated with high plasma levels of one or both of these lipoproteins. Chylomicrons and VLDL carry 150-200 g of triglyceride through the plasma compartment daily, and if mechanisms for their clearance were completely blocked, the plasma triglycerides might rise by more than 4000 mg/dl each day. Therefore their relatively low concentrations in fasting plasma are deceptive, and this is a reflection of their rapid turnover times (Table 15-1). Available evidence suggests that chylomicrons and VLDL are cleared from plasma by a common saturable mechanism.[17] Chylomicrons are preferentially cleared first, and in mild forms of hypertriglyceridemia (plasma triglycerides of 200-500 mg/dl) chylomicrons are rarely found in fasting plasma. When the plasma triglyceride level rises above 700 mg/dl and the diet is not severely fat-restricted, chylomicrons are invariably found. Thus, when hypertriglyceridemia is detected in the fasting plasma of subjects on unrestricted diets, neither observation of chilled plasma nor lipoprotein electrophoresis is necessary to determine which of the triglyceride-rich lipoproteins are elevated. A confident deduction can be made simply from knowledge of the magnitude of the triglyceride elevation.

Low-Density Lipoproteins

Most of the cholesterol in normal plasma is carried in the low-density lipoproteins (LDL). Cholesterol accounts for 50 percent of the weight of LDL (Table 15-2), and simple hypercholesterolemia is synonymous with elevated LDL levels. All available experimental data suggest that no organ or tissue elaborates LDL per se. LDL appear to be the by-products of VLDL catabolism, and hence the predominant cholesterol-rich lipopro-

Table 15-3
Relationship of Plasma Lipid and Lipoprotein Levels

	Potential Variability	Possibly Elevated Cholesterol	Possibly Elevated Triglyceride
VLDL + chylomicrons	~ 100×	Yes	Yes
LDL	~ 3×	Yes	No
HDL	~ 2×	No	No

tein might be viewed as the metabolic garbage remaining after hydrolysis and utilization of VLDL triglyceride. In contrast to VLDL, however, LDL have a distinctly prolonged survival in plasma (Table 15-1). The half-life of LDL in normal subjects is about 3 days, whereas in many hypercholesterolemic subjects it may be 4–5 days.[18] Recent evidence suggests that the LDL complex is removed from plasma by both peripheral tissues and the liver,[19] but the ultimate disposal of the cholesterol eventually must be effected by the liver.

High-Density Lipoproteins

High-density lipoproteins (HDL) contain negligible quantities of triglyceride and only about 20 percent cholesterol (Table 15-2). HDL synthesis by both liver and intestine has been well documented, but nevertheless their functional role is poorly understood. Alterations of HDL content rarely if ever produce hyperlipidemia. HDL levels in women are statistically higher than those in men, and this observation has prompted much speculation that HDL may have a role in removing tissue cholesterol and may account for the apparent protection against atherosclerosis in premenopausal women.[20-22]

TRANSLATION OF HYPERLIPIDEMIA TO HYPERLIPOPROTEINEMIA

Later sections of this chapter will stress that diagnosis and management of hyperlipidemia require only monitoring of the plasma cholesterol and triglyceride levels. Nevertheless, the mental translation of hyperlipidemia to hyperlipoproteinemia can contribute measurably to the intellectual satisfaction and confidence with which these disorders are approached. This translation requires only knowledge of the potential variability of the three major classes of lipoproteins (Table 15-3). Although their content of cholesterol relative to triglyceride is small (Table 15-2), chylomicron and VLDL concentrations can rise to levels 10-fold to 100-fold greater than those normally found, and plasma cholesterol values of several hundred milligrams per deciliter can be demonstrated. Under such circumstances, however, the triglyceride concentration is fourfold to 10-fold greater than that of the cholesterol. Consequently it has become axiomatic that plasma cholesterol levels are not interpretable if the triglyceride concentration is unknown. High levls of LDL alone *never* produce hypertriglyceridemia, and clinically significant elevations of either lipid are not induced by changes in HDL concentration. In the very common clinical situation where moderate hypercholesterolemia and hypertriglyceridemia are found, *both* VLDL and LDL levels are typically increased.

DIAGNOSIS OF HYPERLIPIDEMIA

Sampling

Considering the wide variety of both genetic and acquired disorders that can pathologically elevate blood lipids, every patient, particularly children and young adults, should be screened for hyperlipidemia. Subjects should be encouraged to consume a diet that is normal for their family for at least a week before testing. The quality of the fat and the caloric content of the diet in the few days before sampling can greatly influence both the cholesterol and triglyceride levels. Index or baseline values are most meaningful if drugs known to affect lipid metabolism (and these include birth control pills and conjugated estrogens) are withdrawn 2–4 weeks before sampling is anticipated. Interpretation of laboratory results with respect to both diagnosis and follow-up is greatly facilitated if blood for lipid testing is *always* obtained after at least 12-hr abstinence from fat-containing foods.

Classification of Hyperlipidemia

Measurement of plasma cholesterol and triglyceride is necessary and sufficient to diagnose or exclude hyperlipidemia. When hyperlipidemia is detected, secondary causes, including derangements of thyroid, hepatic and renal function, dysglobulinemia, and diabetic ketoacidosis, must be eliminated. Therapy of the "secondary" hyperlipidemias is always first directed at the primary disorder, but it should be appreciated that hyperlipidemia may be the presenting or dominant clinical feature and may importantly affect the long-term prognosis. In addition, hyperlipidemia associated with diabetes mellitus without ketoacidosis should be considered a primary disorder. Insulin or other therapy of simple hyperglycemia cannot be expected to lower plasma lipids.

With secondary causes of hyperlipidemia eliminated, the hyperlipidemia can be operationally classified as a cholesterol or a triglyceride problem (Table 15–4). Initital therapy is directed exclusively against the offending lipid, and when both cholesterol and triglyceride are elevated, the choice is dictated by the numerically higher lipid. Surprisingly, with this relatively simplistic approach it will rarely be necessary to alter the direction of therapy at a later date.

HYPERCHOLESTROLEMIA

Diet Therapy

Therapy for hyperlipidemia, with or without drugs, almost invariably fails if the patient is unwilling to accept dietary constraints. Moreover, the importances of the various dietary factors that affect the plasma cholesterol level are very widely misunderstood. Diet plans generally stress that the consumption of cholesterol and saturated fat should be limited and the intake of polyunsaturated fats increased. All three factors have been broadly and indiscriminately emphasized, and the conscientious patient has been left utterly bewildered by page after page of dos and don'ts. There is no mischievous intent on the part of the nutritionists and lipidologists who prepare the suggested diets, but the complexities of food and nutrition research have left many pivotal questions unresolved.

Table 15–4
Operational Classification of Hyperlipidemia

Cholesterol problem
   Cholesterol alone elevated
   Cholesterol and triglyceride elevated, but cholesterol greater than triglyceride

Triglyceride problem
   Triglyceride alone elevated
   Triglyceride and cholesterol elevated, but triglyceride greater than cholesterol

It seems evident from a review of most of the published literature on the topic that the importance of limiting cholesterol consumption has been greatly overemphasized. Keys et al.[23] and Mattson et al.,[24] for example, have studied the effects of cholesterol incorporated into formula diets on the plasma cholesterol of volunteers in institutions. They derived equations predicting the influence of dietary cholesterol alterations on the plasma cholesterol (Table 15–5). Their conclusions are somewhat divergent, but they illustrate that radical alterations of cholesterol intake do not profoundly affect plasma cholesterol levels. More recent studies in progress at the National Heart and Lung Institute support this conclusion. The requiem for the egg has been most premature, and we see little justification at present for specifically interdicting intake of eggs or the numberless products made from eggs.

The focus of the cholesterol-lowering diet should therefore revolve around its fat content. The meat and milk of animals and the foodstuffs derived therefrom are the obvious malefactors in the American diet. Their drastic curtailment can produce plasma cholesterol reductions of 50–100 mg/dl in the average patient when coupled with substitution of polyunsaturated fats (Table 15–6). To adequately counsel patients, the physician should be armed with certain general facts concerning the saturated and polyunsaturated fat content of widely used products (Table 15–7). In general, the fat in fowl and fish is considerably less saturated than that in red meat. Some highly saturated fats that may unwittingly be consumed in great quantity include those in milk, butter, coconut, and chocolate (Table 15–7). The vegetable oils that should be recommended are those relatively low in oleic acid content (20–30%) with the higher polyunsaturated/saturated (P/S) ratios. Corn oil is readily available and not very expensive. Safflower oil is more costly, but it has the highest P/S ratio of commercial products. Nutritionists and various diet plans[28–30] can be very helpful in assisting patients in the incorporation of polyunsaturated

Table 15–5
Influence of Dietary Cholesterol on PLasma Cholesterol

Keys[23]
   Δ^* Chol. $= 1.5(\sqrt{\text{Chol.}_i} - \sqrt{\text{Chol.}_f})$†
   $\therefore$ 50% ↓ in dietary Chol. ↓ -7 mg/dl

Mattson[24]
   Δ Chol. $= 0.12 (\text{Chol.}_i - \text{Chol.}_f)$
   $\therefore$ 50% ↓ in dietary Chol. ↓ -20 mg/dl

*Δ = change in plasma cholesterol.
†Chol.$_{i \text{ or } f}$ = milligrams dietary cholesterol/1000 K calories in initial (i) or final (f) diet.

Table 15-6
Effect of Dietary Saturated (S)
and Polyunsaturated (P) Fat on Serum Cholesterol

Keys[25] Δ Chol. $= 2.7\ \Delta S - 1.3\ \Delta P$*
Normal American diet: 40% fat
Normal P/S: 1/3
Fat-modified diet F/S: 2/1

Δ Chol.† $= 2.7\ (13-30) - 1.3\ (27-10)$
　　　　$= -68$ mg/dl

*S and P are percentages of total calories.
†This calculation is oversimplified, ignoring the relatively high ($\geq 30\%$) diet content of monounsaturated fat.

Table 15-7
Fat Content of Various Foods*

	% Fat	% Oleic Acid	~P/S†
Meats (raw)			
Bacon	55	50	0.3
Beef	11	49	0.1
Chicken	13	45	0.6
Duck	29	49	0.9
Lamb	18	39	0.1
Pork	25	43	0.2
Dairy			
Egg‡	11	38	0.4
Milk (whole)	4	29	0.1
Butter	81	29	0.1
Oils			
Coconut	100	6	0.2
Olive	100	77	4.3
Peanut	100	51	9.7
Cottonseed	100	24	15.0
Corn	100	30	28.0
Soybean	100	27	34.5
Sunflower	100	24	39.0
Safflower	100	19	78.9
Other			
Avocado	27	63	0.7
Chocolate (unsweetened)	54	36	0.0
Cocoa (powder)	24	36	0.0
Nuts (most)	~50	~50	1-3
Walnuts	58	22	7.6

*Calculated from data of Harcinge and Crooks.[26]
†P/S = polyunsaturated/saturated fat ratio.
‡Calculated from data of Posati et al.[27]

fats in their diets. Nevertheless, the greatest impediment to successful diet therapy is the reluctance of many patients to radically limit their red meat consumption.

The message to the patient can be succinctly stated: The key factor in the diet is reduction of saturated fat consumption. You can eat red meat (i.e., lamb, pork, or beef) once or twice a week, but trim all visible fat. The rest of the time eat skinned defatted chicken, fish, or eggs. Do not eat cheese, only cheese substitutes. Drink nonfat milk; the 1% and 2% forms are no good. Do not eat ice cream or ice milk or butter. Use soft tub margarine or mayonnaise as a spread; use liberal amounts of corn or safflower oil for cooking and salads, and do not eat anything cooked in lard or regular shortening. You can cheat 1 day every 2 weeks. Plan that day. The rest of the time be very strict. If you cheat just a little every day, you will see very little lowering of your blood cholesterol.

Drug Therapy

Drug therapy, in addition to diet, is frequently necessary in the relatively uncommon disease of familial hypercholesterolemia with xanthomatosis and in the many other forms of moderate hypercholesterolemia of diverse etiology.

Some pharmacologic and clinical information on the three most effective drugs is included for reference (Table 15–8). The nonabsorbable bile acid sequestrant cholestyramine is the drug of first choice. It should be recognized that acute administration of large doses (24–32 g/day) can produce a bowel obstruction syndrome. When the drug is chronically prescribed, it is usually necessary to employ stool softeners with or without mild laxatives. Malabsorption of fat and fat-soluble vitamins occurs only infrequently and with daily doses greater than 20 g.

Nicotinic acid is a good second-line drug that is less expensive and is also quite effective in combination with cholestyramine. Patient acceptance is much improved if very small doses are used initially and if the medication is taken after meals. The chemical and symptomatic side effects of the drug (Table 15–8) have discouraged its general use, but they have proved limiting in very few patients in our clinic.

Dextrothyroxine should probably be employed only in younger patients without clinical evidence of coronary heart disease. As recommended by others,[31] we use dextrothyroxine in combination with propranolol in patients with symptomatic coronary disease. Because of the findings of the Coronary Drug Project,[32] however, the potential risks and gains must be carefully weighed in such cases.

All three of these drugs can potentially reduce plasma cholesterol by 20% or more, and there is no evidence that their hypolipidemic effects diminish with prolonged therapy. Secondary failures are not uncommon in treating lipid disorders, but they are attributable to poor dietary adherence, not drug tachyphylaxis.

HYPERTRIGLYCERIDEMIA

Diet Therapy

If the hypertriglyceridemic patient is obese, caloric restriction is the only therapy necessary. Triglyceride levels will fall dramatically when calories are reduced, even before measurable weight loss is demonstrable, and the effect will be sustained for a lifetime if ideal body weight can be achieved. Another selected group of patients can

Table 15–8
Drugs for Hypercholesterolemia

	Cholestyramine	Nicotinic Acid	D-Thyroxine
Brand name	Questran	Lipo-Nicin, Nicolar, Nicobid (niacin)	Choloxin
Mechanism	Bile acid sequestrant	↓ FFA release, others	↑ cholesterol excretion, others
Effect on plasma lipoproteins	↑ LDL Catabolism; ↓ LDL level; may ↑ VLDL	↓ VLDL synthesis; ↓ VLDL + LDL levels	?↑ LDL catabolism; ↓ LDL level
Initial dose	4 g p.o. t.i.d.	100 mg p.o. t.i.d.	2 mg p.o. q.d.
Maintenance dose	16–32 g q.d.	3–6 g q.d.	4–8 q.d.
Adverse effects*	Constipation, bloating, nausea, vomiting, abdominal pain, fat malabsorption (at high doses)	Flushing, itching, acanthosis nigricans, abnormal LFTs, hyperglycemia, hyperuricemia, jaundice, cirrhosis	Hypermetabolism, ↑ angina, ?↑ coronary death rate
Drug–drug interactions	Binds many drugs: warfarin, digitalis, thyroxine, phenylbutazone, chlorothiazide, tetracycline and others (including fat-soluble vitamins)	None	Potentiates warfarin
Cost/month	$30–$60	$7–$10	$12–$15

*See PDR for other side effects.

return to normal chemistries if they limit their ethanol consumption to modest quantities on social occasions.

The advantage of restricting either total caloric fat or carbohydrate in treating hypertriglyceridemia has been overstated. Fat restriction is important only in the face of massive hypertriglyceridemia with the concomitant risk of precipitating life-threatening pancreatitis. In such patients the abrupt withdrawal of dietary fat will lower the plasma triglycerides by several thousand milligrams per deciliter in 2–3 days.

There is little convincing evidence that restricting dietary carbohydrate has a role in the management of any form of hypertriglyceridemia. It is well known that feeding large quantities of carbohydrate can double the plasma triglyceride level in both normals and hypertriglyceridemics, and this observation has given support to the notion of "carbohydrate-sensitive" hypertriglyceridemia. However, such induced hypertriglyceridemia spontaneously resolves when high-carbohydrate diets are continued for prolonged periods. Finally, if both dietary fat and carbohydrate are restricted, protein must eventually be substituted to maintain caloric balance. High-protein diets are not palatable. In the long term, almost all hypertriglyceridemic subjects are maintained on essentially balanced diets with restriction only of total calories and alcohol.

Drug Therapy

The lean patient with hypertriglyceridemia usually requires drug therapy. Clofibrate (Atromid-S) should be tried first because of the very low incidence of troublesome side effects attending its use. It is most likely to be effective in mild to moderate hypertriglyceridemia (triglycerides = 300–700 mg/dl). If the plasma triglyceride concentration exceeds 1000 mg/dl, a significant therapeutic effect from clofibrate should not be expected. Nicotinic acid is the drug of choice in severe hypertriglyceridemia, with cautious dose increases as recommended for hypercholesterolemia (Table 15–8). In contrast to the treatment of hypercholesterolemia, however, low doses (1.5–3.0 g/day) will often produce satisfactory control of hypertriglyceridemia. Again, it must be emphasized that drug therapy does not obviate the need for rigorous dietary prescription.

LIPOPROTEIN ELECTROPHORESIS AND LIPOPROTEIN PHENOTYPING

The schema for the diagnosis and management of the hyperlipidemias developed herein has purposely been developed outside the constructs of the Fredrickson-Levy-Lees classification system.[33] There is little doubt that their typing system will be employed for many more years, but its clinical relevance has undergone rapid evolution, and much of the confusion in the current medical literature has its genesis in the interpretation of what the typing system connoted. The Fredrickson-Levy-Lees types were too often construed as specific diseases, usually familial. It is not difficult to identify the genesis of this confusion. The typing system emerged from studies of a very unique referral population composed of patients with the severest abnormalities. For the most part they not only had familial hyperlipidemia, but monogenic hyperlipidemia as well. This led to the definition of unambiguous "diagnostic" categories with little overlap. Subsequent experience in many other clinics has shown that the apparent "type" of hyperlipoproteinemia is anything but immutable. Type V hyperlipoproteinemia (elevated chylomicrons and VLDL) can convert to type IV hyperlipoproteiemia (elevated VLDL) with no specific treatment. Patients may fulfill criteria for type IV (elevated VLDL) on one occasion and type IIb (elevated VLDL and LDL) on another. In addition, a perplexing variety of "types" can occur unpredictably, often in a single family. It became painfully obvious that a hyperlipoproteinemic "type" could not be confidently equated with a disease, familial or acquired.

It was also most unfortunate that lipoprotein electrophoresis came to be regarded as the necessary and sufficient tool to perform "lipoprotein phenotyping." Preparative ultracentrifugation, *not* lipoprotein electrophoresis, was the primary laboratory technique in the design of the original typing system. And there is no evidence that lipoprotein electrophoresis, without preparative ultracentrifugation, contributes useful information not provided by simple measurement of plasma cholesterol and triglyceride levels.[34,35]

What is the status of the typing system today? The "types" still provide an accurate and almost inclusive shorthand nomenclature for describing virtually all possible patterns of plasma lipoprotein elevations encountered clinically. Their use very economically facilitates written and oral communication between researchers, but they serve as little more than window dressing in the private patient's chart.

REFERENCES

1. Keys A, Kimura N, Kusukawa A, et al: Lessons from serum cholesterol studies in Japan, Hawaii and Los Angeles. Ann Intern Med 48:83, 1958
2. Chapman JM, Massey FJ JR: The interrelationships of serum cholesterol, hypertension, body weight, and risk of coronary disease. Results of the first ten years' follow-up in the Los Angeles Heart Study. J Chronic Dis 17:933, 1964
3. Keys A (ed): Coronary heart disease in seven countries. Circulation 41 [Suppl I]:1, 1970
4. Kannel WB: Serum cholesterol, lipoproteins, and the risk of coronary heart disease. The Framingham study. Ann Intern Med 74:1, 1971
5. Armstrong ML, Warner ED, Connor WE: Regression of coronary atheromatosis in rhesus monkeys. Circ Res 27:59, 1970
6. Hollander W, Kramsch DM: The distribution of intravenously administered ^{3}H-cholesterol in arteries and other tissues. J Atheroscler Res 7:491, 1967
7. Scott PJ, Hurley PJ: The distribution of radioiodinated albumin and low density lipoprotein in tissues and the artery wall. Atherosclerosis 11:77, 1970
8. Getz GS, Vesselinovitch D, Wissler RW: A dynamic pathology of atherosclerosis. Am J Med 46:657, 1969
9. Porter R, Knight J: Atherogenesis: Initiating Factors. Amsterdam, Associated Scientific, 1973
10. Wissler RW: Development of the atherosclerotic plaque, *in* Braunwald E (ed): The Myocardium: Failure and Infarction. New York, H. P. Publishing, 1974, p 155
11. Fasman GD (ed): Handbook of Biochemistry and Molecular Biology (ed 3). Cleveland, CRC Press, 1975, p 486
12. Bronte-Stewart B, Antonis A, Eales L, et al: Effects of feeding different fats on serum-cholesterol levels. Lancet 1:522, 1956
13. Ahrens EH Jr, Hirsch J, Insull W Jr, et al: The influence of dietary fats on serum lipid levels in man. Lancet 1:943, 1957
14. Keys A, Anderson JT, Grande F: Serum cholesterol response to changes in the diet. IV. Particular saturated fatty acids in the diet. Metabolism 14:776, 1965
15. Connor WH, Stone DB, Hodges RE: The interrelated effects of dietary cholesterol and fat upon human serum lipid levels. J Clin Invest 43 1691, 1964
16. Dietschy JM, Wilson JD: Regulation of cholesterol metabolism. N Engl J Med 282:1128, 1970
17. Brunzell JD, Hazzard WR, Porte D Jr, et al: Evidence for a common, saturable, triglyceride removal mechanism for chylomicrons and very low density lipoproteins in man. J Clin Invest 52:1578, 1973
18. Langer T, Strober W, Levy RI: The metabolism of low density lipoprotein in familial type II hyperlipoproteinemia. J Clin Invest 51:1528, 1972
19. Sniderman AD, Carew TE, Chandler JG, et al: Paradoxical increase in rate of catabolism of

low-density lipoproteins after hepatectomy. Science 183:526, 1974
20. Miller GJ, Miller NE: Plasma high-density lipoprotein concentration and development of ischaemic heart disease. Lancet 1:16, 1975
21. Hsia SL, Hennekens CH, Chao Yu-S, et al: Decreased serum cholesterol-ginding reserve in premature myocardial infarction. Lancet 2:1000, 1975
22. Rhoads GG, Gulbrandsen CL, Kagan A: Serum lipoproteins and coronary heart disease in a population study of Hawaii Japanese men. N Engl J Med 294:293, 1976
23. Keys A, Anderson JT, Grande F: Serum cholesterol response to changes in the diet. II. The effect of cholesterol in the diet. Metabolism 14:759, 1965
24. Mattson FH, Erickson BA, Kligman AM: Effect of dietary cholesterol on serum cholesterol in man. Am J Clin Nutr 25:589, 1972
25. Keys A, Anderson JT, Grande F: Serum cholesterol response to changes in the diet. I. Iodine value of dietary fat versus 2S-P. Metabolism 14:747, 1965
26. Hardinge MG, Crooks H: Fatty acid composition of food fats. J AM Diet Assoc 34:1065, 1958
27. Posati LP, Kinsella JE, Watt BK: The fatty acid composition of milk and eggs — provisional tables. Presented at 57th Annual Meeting, American Dietetic Association, Philadelphia, Oct 7–11, 1974
28. Keys, A, Keys M: Eat and stay well. Garden City, NY, Doubleday, 1963
29. Low Fat and Vegetable Oil Recipes. Cleveland Clinic Research Division, 2020 East 93rd St, Cleveland, Ohio
30. Havenstein N, Richardson E: The Anti-coronary Cookbook. New York, Grosset & Dunlap, 1971
31. Krikler DM, Lefevre D, Lewis B: Dextrothyroxine with propranolol in treatment of hypercholesterolemia. Lancet 1:934, 1971
32. Coronary Drug Project: Findings leading to further modifications of its protocol with respect to dextrothyroxine. JAMA 220:996, 1972
33. Fredrickson DS, Levy RI, Lees RS: Fat transport in lipoproteins—an integrated approach to mechanisms and disorders. N Engl J Med 276:32, 1967
34. Fredrickson DS: It's time to be practical. Circulation 51:209, 1975
35. Iammarino RM: Lipoprotein electrophoresis should be discontinued as a routine procedure. Clin Chem 21:300, 1975

Index

Achilles reflex, hypothyroidism, 22, 32
Acne vulgaris, 88
ACTH (adrenocorticotropic hormone), 49
  deficiencies, 50
  pituitary ACTH reserve, 52
  rapid test with plasma aldosterone levels, 54
  standard intravenous ACTH testing, 51–52
    abnormal response to, 52
  stimulation of aldosterone secretion, 52, 73
  24-hr infusion test, 90, 94–95
Addison's disease, 49, 50–53
  chronic adrenocortical insufficiency, 50
  symptoms, 50
  treatment, 53
Adenomas
  adrenocortical, 57, 65
  hypercortisolism, 67–68
  pituitary, 57, 65
Adrenal atrophy, 49–50, 52
Adrenal cortex, 49, 73
Adrenal crisis, 50
  adrenocortical insufficiency, 50
  treatment, 53–54
Adrenal hyperplasia syndrome, 49
  bilateral, 57, 65–67
Adrenocortical insufficiency, 49–55
  ACTH testing, 51–52
  chronic, 50
  diagnosis, 49–51
  education of patients, 53
  etiologies, 49–50
  plasma cortisol response following cosyntropin, 50–51
  primary (Addison's disease), 49, 51, 53
  secondary, 49, 50, 51
  symptoms of hypofunction, 51
  therapy, 51–54

Alcoholic ketoacidosis, 131
Aldosterone
  control mechanisms for release of, 73–74
  isolated deficiency, 54
  plasma renin activity and, 85
  secretion following ACTH stimulation, 49, 51, 52
  volume and potassium feedback loops, 74–75
Aldosteronism
  diagnosis, 84
  hypertension and hyperaldosteronism, 76
  primary, 79–80, 84
  renin-aldosterone volume control loop, 76
  screening procedures, 79–80
Aminocentesis, 143
Androgens, 49
  decreased serum TBG, 6
  doses, 53
Anemia, pernicious, 23, 24
Angiotensin II, 74
  adrenal response to, 78–79
Ankle reflexes, hypothyroidism, 20
Anterior pituitary hypothyroidism, 4
Antithyroid agents and hypothyroidism, 27–28
Atherosclerosis, 153, 155, 158
  atherogenesis, 23
Azotemia, 50, 145

Basal metabolic rate (BMR), 7
  hypothyroidism, 32
  tests of actions of thyroid hormones, 15
Beta-adrenergic blocking agents, 15

Bicarbonate in diabetic ketoacidosis therapy, 134–135
Bilateral adrenocortical hyperplasia, 49, 57, 65–67
Biochemical changes, hypothyroidism, 29–32
Blindness, caused by diabetic retinopathy, 147

Calcium urolithiasis, 98–99
   control of, 102
Carcinoma
   adrenal, 57
   adrenocortical, 65
   pituitary, 65
Cardiovascular-pulmonary system
   hyperlipidemia and, 153, 160
   hypothyroidism and, 22–23
Carpal tunnel syndrome, 22
Catecholamines, in thyroid hormone actions, 15
Children and infants
   of diabetic mothers, 144–145
   fetal thyroid, 28
   hypercortisolism, 58
   hypothyroidism, 20, 29
Cholesterol, 155–157
   biosynthesis, 155–156
   diet therapy, 159–162
   fat content of various foods, 161–162
   hypercholstrolemia, 159–162
   hypothyroidism, 24
   influence of dietary cholesterol on plasma cholesterol, 154, 160
   lipoprotein composition, 157–158
   low-density lipoproteins, 157–158
Cholestyramine for hypercholesterolemia, 162–163
Chronic autoimmune thyroiditis (Hashimoto's disease), 25–26, 49–50
Chylomicrons and VLDL, 157
Cirrhosis, decreased serum TBG, 6
Clinical appraisal of patient, 7
   history and physical examination, 7
   laboratory tests of thyroid function, 7–15
Cold intolerance, hypothyroidism, 20, 21
Coma, hypothyroidism, 21–22
Congeners, thyroid hormone, 15
Corticosteroids, effect on carbohydrate intolerance, 111

Cortisol. *See also* Glucocorticoids
   ACTH testing, 51–52
   and aldosterone responses after cosyntropin, 53–54
   Cushing's syndrome, 57–71
   dexamethasone suppression tests, 60–63
   diabetes and pregnancy, 139
   diagnostic tests, 64–65
   hypercortisolism, 65–69
   hypothyroidism, 24
   laboratory tests
      plasma cortisol concentrations, 59–60
      urinary 17-OCHS per gram of creatinine, 58
   plasma concentrations, 59–60
   secretion rate, 58, 63–64
   tests for adrenal insufficiency, 50–51
   urinary excretion, 57–58, 63
Cortisone
   primary adrenocortical insufficiency therapy, 53
   -primed oral glucose tolerance tests, 115
Cortrosyn, ACTH 24-hr infusion test, 90, 94–95
   interpretation, 94–95
   procedures, 94
Cosyntropin
   plasma aldosterone responses, 50–51, 53
   plasma cortisol responses, 53
Creatine phosphokinase, 22
Creatinine, urinary 17-OHCS per gram of creatinine test, 58
Cushing's syndrome, 57–71
   in children, 58
   definition, 57
   diagnosis, 57–58
      comparison of tests, 64–65
   hypercortisolism
      athologic diagnosis, 65–67
      treatment of, 67–69
   laboratory procedures, 58–65
      cortisol secretion rate, 63–64
      dexamethasone suppression tests, 60–63
      plasma cortisol concentration, 59–60
      urinary excretion of free cortisol, 63
      urinary 17-OHCS per gram of creatinine, 58
   screening procedures, 57
   signs and symptoms, 57–59
   treatment, 57–58

Index

Dexamethasone suppression tests, 60–63
  overnight, 60–61
  two-day test
    of Liddle, 61–62
    modified, 62
  2-mg test, 89–90, 93
    differentiating tumors and bilateral adrenal hyperplasia, 66–68
    to rule out Cushing's syndrome, 93
Dextrothyroxine with propranolol in hypercholesterolemia, 162–163
Diabetes mellitus, 107–151
  gestational, 137–139, 142
  glucose tolerance testing. *See* Oral glucose tolerance testing
  hyperlipidemia without ketoacidosis, 159
  juvenile-onset diabetics, 119
    retinopathy, 147
  ketoacidosis. *See* Ketoacidosis, diabetic
  maturity-onset, 125, 127
  in offspring of two diabetic parents, 118–119
  oral glucose tolerance testing, 107–124. *See also* Oral glucose tolerance testing
  oral hypoglycemic drugs, 125–126
    contraindications, 125–126
    phenformin, 126–127, 128
    risk factors, 125
    sulfonylureas, 126–127
  pregnancy complicated by, 137–146
    classification of, 140–141
    delivery, 144
    effect on maternal diabetes, 145
    gestational diabetes, 137–139, 142
    management of, 141–143
    management of newborn, 144–145
    maternal complications, 142–143
    metabolic changes in pregnancy, 138–139
    prediabetics, 137
    risk factors, 139–140
    screening procedures, 139–140
  retinopathy, 145, 147–151. *See also* Retinopathy, diabetic
  symptomatic, 119
  therapy, 125–128
    calorie control and/or body weight control, 125
    diet, 125, 127
    insulin, 127
    risk factors, 125
    sulfonylureas, 126–127
    tolbutamide, 126
    University Group Diabetes Program (UGDP), 125–128
Diabetic ketoacidosis, 129–135
  diagnosis, 131
    nitroprusside reaction, 131
  insulin therapy, 132–134
    administration, 132–134
    choice of regimen, 133–134
    physiology, 132
  ketone production, 130–131
  pathogenesis, 129–131
    hyperglycemia, 129–130
    metabolic acidosis, 130–131
  treatment, 131–135
Diabetic Retinopathy Study, 150
Diabetic Retinopathy Vitrectomy Study, 150
Diiodotyrosine (DIT), 3
Diphenylhydantoin preparations, 88, 111
Diphosphonates, in renal hypercalciurias, 105–106
D-thyroxine (Choloxin), 13

Edema
  hypothyroidism, 20–21
  mucinous, 19
  periorbital, 20–21
Electrocardiograms, hypothyroidism, 22
Electrolysis, for hirsute females, 87, 91
Energy metabolism, hypothyroidism, 23–24
Enzyme deficiencies
  partial 11- or 21-hydroxylase, 90, 91, 95
Epinephrine, relationship to thyroid hormones, 15
Estriol, monitoring fetal well-being, 143
Estrogen
  diabetes and pregnancy, 138
  increased serum TBG and, 6

Fat content of various foods, 161–162
Fatty acids, 153–154
  monounsaturated, 154–155

Fatty acids, *continued*
　　polyunsaturated, 154–155
　　saturated, 154–155
　　transport of, 154–155
Fluid treatment, diabetic ketoacidosis, 131–132
Fluorohydrocortisone, 53
Free thyroxine (FT4), 2
　　method of calculating, 13
Free triiodothyronine (FT3), 2
Furosemide, test for low-renin hypertension, 77

Gas-liquid chromatographic methods for measuring T3, 38
Gastrointestinal system, effects of hypothyroidism, 23
Glaucoma, neovascular, 149
Glucagon, levels during pregnancy, 139
Glucocorticoids, 49
　decreased serum TBG, 6
　insufficiency, 50
　replacement intake, 53–54
Glucose
　hyperglycemia, 129–130
　intolerance in high-risk patients, 118
Glutamic oxaloacetic transaminase, 22
Goetsch test, thyroid hormone functions, 15
Goiters
　hypothyroidism and, 4–5, 28
　　acquired, 4
　　chronic lymphoid (Hashimoto's), 5
　　drug-induced, 4
　　hereditary, 4
　　iodide myxedema, 4
　　nodular with T3 secretion, 4
　　toxic multinodular, 40
Granulomatous disorders, 4–5
Graves' disease, 4, 26–27
　T3 toxicosis, 40
Growth hormone secretion
　hypothyroidism, 24–25
　during pregnancy, 139

Hand-Schüller-Christian disease, 28
Hashimoto's disease (chronic autoimmune thyroiditis), 4–5, 25–26, 40
　idiopathic primary adrenal insufficiency and, 49–50
"Hashitoxicosis" with hypothyroidism, 13
Hematopoietic system, effect of hypothyroidism, 24
Hirsutism in females, 87–95
　causes, 88
　definition, 87
　differentiating from virilism, 88–89
　electrolysis, 87, 91
　idiopathic, 91
　laboratory studies, 89–90
　　ACTH 24-hr infusion test, 90
　　inpatient, 90–91
　　laparoscopy, 90–91
　　outpatient, 89–90
　　partial adrenogenital syndrome, 90
　　serum luteinizing hormone (LH), 89
　　serum testosterone, 89
　　standard 2-mg dexamethasone suppression tests, 89–90
　outpatient evaluation, 87–89
　　history and physical examination, 87–89
　　menstrual irregularities, 88
　partial adrenogenital syndrome, 90–91
　Stein-Leventhal Syndrome, 91
　therapy, 91
Human chorionic gonadotropin, 143
Human placental lactogen (HPL), 138–139, 143
Hydramnios, 142–143
11- or 21-hydroxylation deficiency, 90–91
Hyperaldosteronism
　hypertension and, 76
　screening procedures, 79–80
Hypercalciurias, 98–106
　absorptive, 98–99
　causes of, 98–99
　diagnostic criteria, 99–102
　idiopathic, 98
　primary hyperparathyroidism, 99–100
　renal, 98
　resorptive, 98
　therapeutic considerations, 102–106
　　diphosphonates, 105–106
　　orthophosphates, 103–105
　　sodium cellulose phosphate, 102–103
　　thiazides, 105
　urinary cyclic AMP, 101
Hypercholestrolemia, 23, 157–162

Index

diet therapy, 159–162
drug therapy, 162–163
  cholestyramine, 162–163
  dextrothyoxine with propranolol, 162–163
  nicotinic acid, 162–163
familial, 162
Hypercortisolism, 58, 65–69
  pathologic diagnosis, 65–67
  treatment, 67–69
Hyperglycemia, 126–127, 159
  diabetic ketoacidosis, 129–130
Hyperkalemia, 50
  hypoaldosterone syndromes, 54
Hyperketonemia, 130–131
Hyperlipidemia
  cholesterol problem, 159–160
  classification of, 159–160
  coronary heart disease and, 153
  diagnosis, 153, 159
  lipids, 153–157
    cholesterol, 155–157
    fatty acids, 153–154
    triglycerides, 154–155
  screening for, 159
  translation to hyperlipoproteinemia, 158
  triglyceride problem, 159–160
  typing system, 164–165
    Frederickson-Levy-Lees types, 164–165
Hyperlipoproteinemia, 153–166
  diagnosis of hyperlipidemia, 159
    classification of, 159–160
    screening for, 159
  fat content of various foods, 161–162
  hypercholestrolemia, 159–162
  hypertriglyceridemia, 162–163
  lipids, 153–157
    cholesterol, 155–157
    fatty acids, 153–154
    triglyceride, 154–155
  lipoprotein electrophoresis and lipoprotein phenotyping, 164–165
  plasma lipoproteins, 157–158
    chylomicrons and VLDL, 157
    high-density lipoproteins, 158
    low-density lipoproteins, 157–158
  translation of hyperlipidemia to, 158
Hyperosmolarity, 129–130
Hyperparathyroidism, 98
Hypertension
  clinical evaluation of patient, 83–85

hyperaldosteronism and, 76
low-renin, 78–79
plasma renin activity and aldosterone, 85
renin-angiotensin-aldosterone axis and, 73–81
screening procedures for primary aldosteronism, 79–80
serum and urinary potassium, 84–85
sodium loading test, 85
women and blacks, 77
Hyperthyroidism, 3
  borderline, 40
  clinical laboratory tests, 12
  with normal T3 levels, 43–44
  thyroid function tests, 12
  T3 toxicosis and, 37–47
Hypertrichosis, 88
Hypertriglyceridemia, 23, 157, 158, 162–164
  diet therapy, 162–164
  drug therapy, 164
Hypoaldosterone syndromes, 54
  diagnosis of, 54
  hyponatremia and hyperkalemia, 54
  isolated, 49
Hypoglycemia, 52
  during pregnancy, 142
  reactive, 120–122
    blood glucose and serum insulin levels, 122
    incidence, 121
    oral glucose tolerance testing, 120–122
    symptoms, 120
Hyponatremia, 50, 54
Hypoparathyroidism, 50
Hyporeninism, 54
Hypothalamic hypothyroidism, 4–5
Hypothalamic-pituitary ACTH deficiency, 49
Hypothalamic/pituitary/thyroid gland axis, 1
  thyroid function tests 8–13
  TRH/TSH short-loop activity, 2
Hypothyroidism, 19–35
  biochemical manifestations and laboratory tests, 29–32
  causes, 20, 25–29
    hypothyrotropic hypothyroidism, 28–29
    loss of functional thyroid tissue, 25–27
      chronic autoimmune thyroiditis, 26
      following thyroidectomy, 26–27
      idiopathic hypothyroidism, 25–26
      ^{131}I therapy, 26
      thyroid dysgenesis, 27

Hypothyroidism, *continued*
    transient hypothyroidism, 27
    peripheral resistance to thyroid hormones, 29
    thyroid biosynthetic defects, 27–28
        antithyroid agents, 27–28
        inherited defects, 27
        iodine deficiency, 27
  definition of, 19
  diagnosis of, 19–32
  differential aspects of, 5
  etiologies of, 4
  goitrous, 4
  acquired, 4
    chronic lymphoid (Hashimoto's) thyroiditis, 5
    drug-induced, 4
    hereditary, 4
    iodide myxedema, 4
  "hashitoxicosis" with, 5, 13
  hypothalamic, 4–5
  hypothyrotropic, 28–29
    differentiation from thyroidal, 30
    TRH deficiency, 28–29
    TSH deficiency, 28
  idiopathic (atrophic thyroiditis), 4, 24–26
  infantile, 29
  laboratory tests for, 9, 12–13
    outline for evaluation of patients, 31–32
  manifestations of, 19–25
    cardiovascular-pulmonary system, 22–23
    endocrine system, 24–25
    energy metabolism, 23–24
    gastrointestinal system, 23
    hematopoietic system, 24
    musculoskeletal system, 22
    nervous system, 21–22
    physical appearance, 20–21
    renal function, 23
    skin and appendages, 21
    symptoms and signs, 25
  myxedema, 4, 19
  nongoitrous, 4
  with normal T3 levels, 43
  postoperative, 4
  postradiation, 4
  primary, 4–5
  secondary, 4–5
    anterior pituitary, 4
    hypothalamic hypothyroidism, 4
  therapy for, 32–33
    dosage, 32–33
    preparations for, 33
  thyroid function tests, 9–12

Insulin therapy
  administration, 132–133
  diabetic ketoacidosis, 131, 132–134
  hypothyroidism, 24
  low-dose continuous infusion technique, 133
  physiology, 132
  pregnancy and diabetes, 138–139
  regimen, choice of, 133–134
  secretory rates, 132
  tolerance testing, 52
  turnover rates, 132
Iodides
  metabolism, 3
  myxedema, 4, 19
Iodine deficiency
  hypothyroidism and, 25, 27
  T3 toxicosis and, 41–42
Iron deficiency, 24

Ketoacidosis, diabetic, 129–135
  diagnosis of, 131
    nitroprusside reaction, 131
  hyperlipidemia without ketoacidosis, 159
  insulin deficiency, 129
  insulin therapy, 132–134
    administration, 132–133
    choice of regimen, 133–134
    low-dose continuous infusion technique, 133–134
    physiology, 132
  ketone production, 130–131
  mortality rate, 129
  pathogenesis, 129–131
    hyperglycemia, 129–130
    metabolic acidosis, 130–131
  during pregnancy, 142
  treatment, 131–135
Kidney stones. *See* Renal stones

Index

Laboratory procedures
  in Cushing's syndrome, 58–65
    cortisol secretion rate, 63–64
    dexamethasone suppression tests, 60–63
    plasma cortisol concentration, 59–60
    urinary excretion of free cortisol, 63
    urinary 17-OHCS per gram of creatinine, 58
  dexamethasone suppression tests, 60–63, 66–68
    overnight, 60–61
    two-day test
      of Liddle, 61–62
      modified, 62
    2-mg, 89–90, 93
  discordant serum T4:T3 ratios, 11
  hirsutism, 89–90
    ACTH 24-hr infusion test, 90
    dexamethasone suppression test, 89–90, 93
    laparoscopy, 90–91
    partial adrenogenital syndrome, 90
    serum luteinizing hormone, 89
    serum testosterone, 89
  hyperthyroidism, 12
  hypothalamic/pituitary/thyroid function, 8–13
  hypothyroidism, 9–12, 29–32
    antithyroid antibodies test, 32
    competitive protein binding analysis (T4-D), 29
    low serum T4 concentration (T4-RIA), 29
    serum T3 resin uptake tests, 29
    serum TSH concentration, 30
    serum TSH responses to TRH, 30–31
    thyroidal ^{131}I uptake test, 32
  physiologic precepts for evaluating, 1–17
  thyroid function, 7–15
    circulating thyroid hormone levels, 8, 13–15
    hypothalamic/pituitary/thyroid relationship, 8–13
    tissue oxidative metabolism, 8, 15
  thyroid hormone transport in the circulation, 13–15
    peripheral action, 15
    serum total T3 and FT3 concentrations, 14
    serum total T4 and free T4, 13–14
    tissue oxidative metabolism, 8, 15
    basal metabolic rate, 15
Lactic acidosis, 126
Lactic dehydrogenase, 22
Laparoscopy, hirsute women, 90–91
Lecithin/sphingomyelin ratio, 143
Leukocyte antigens, 50
Linoleic acid, 154–155
Lipids, 153–157
  cholesterol, 155–157
  fatty acids, 153–154
  triglyceride, 154–155
Lipoproteins, 156–158
  composition, 157
  electrophoresis, 164–165
  high-density, 158
  hyperlipoproteinemia. *See* Hyperlipoproteinemia
  low-density, 157–158
  phenotyping, 164–165
  plasma, 156–158
    chylomicrons and VLDL, 157
  relationship of plasma lipid and lipoprotein levels, 158
  very low density (VLDL), 157
Lithium carbonate, antithyroid effects, 28

Macular edema, diabetic retinopathy, 149
Malnutrition, decreased serum TBG, 6
Melanocyte-stimulating hormone, 50
Melanosis, 50
Metabolic acidosis, 130–131
Metabolic alkalosis, 134
Metabolites, thyroid hormone, 14
Methimazole, antithyroid effects, 28
Metyrapone (Metopirone) tests, 52, 66, 68
Mineralocorticoids, 49
  replacement therapy, 52–54
Moniliasis, 50
Monoiodotyrosine (MIT), 3
Musculoskeletal system, effect of hypothyroidism, 22
Myxedema, 4, 19

Nephrolithiasis, 97
Nephrosis, decreased serum TBG, 6

Nervous system, effect of hypothyroidism, 21–22
Nicotinic acid
  for hypercholesterolemia, 162–163
  for hypertriglyceridemia, 164
Nitroprusside tablets (Acetest), 131

Oral contraceptive agents, effect on carbohydrates, 111
Oral glucose tolerance testing, 107–124
  blood glucose levels and plasma glucose levels, 111
  chemical diabetes, 116, 118
  cortisone-primed oral glucose tolerance tests, 115
  detection of carbohydrate intolerance, 107, 111
  dose administrations, 107–108
  factors influencing results, 108–111
    age, 110
    drug history, 111
    endocrine status, 110–111
    obesity, 108
    physical activity, 110
  family studies, 118–119
  hypothyroidism, 23–24
  implications, 107–124
  intolerance in high-risk patients, 118
  interpretations in outpatients, 111
  intravenous and, 107
  meaning of mildly abnormal results, 116–118
  offspring of two diabetic parents, 115–120
    risk of developing diabetes, 120
  preparation diet, 108–110
  prior steroid administration, 115
  reactive hypoglycemia, 114, 120–122
    blood glucose and serum insulin relationship, 122
  reproducibility, 116–117
  sex differences, 113–114
  test standardization, 108
  upper limits of normal, 111–115
Orthophosphates, for renal calculi, 103–105
Oxygen spirometry, diagnosis of thyrotoxicosis, 15
Oxytocin challenge test with fetal monitoring, 143

Palmitic acid, 154
Paresthesias, hypothyroidism, 20, 22
Parathyroid hormone, 98
Partial adrenogenital syndrome, 90–91
Phenformin, 126–128
  contraindications for, 126
Phenothiazines, 88
Phosphates in renal hypercalciurias, 102–106
Phospholipids, lipoprotein composition, 157
Photocoagulation treatment, 149–150
Pituitary disease, 28
  serum TSH concentrations, 30
Pituitary glands
  ablation, 150
  ACTH reserve, 52
  adenomas or carcinomas, 57, 65
  hypothyroidism and, 24
  idiopathic failure, 5
  ischemic necrosis (Sheehan's syndrome), 4–5, 28
  secondary hypothyroidism, 4
  tropic hormone deficiencies, 50
Pituitary stalk section, hypothalamic hypothyroidism, 4
Plummer's disease, 4
Potassium
  hypertension, 84–85
  renin-angiotensin-aldosterone system and, 73–76
  treatment of diabetic ketoacidosis, 134
Prednisone
  adrenocortical insufficiency therapy, 53
  partial adrenogenital syndrome, 91
Preeclampsia, 142–143
Pregnancy and diabetes, 137–146
  adult-onset diabetes, 138
  classification, 140–141
  delivery, 144
    deciding time for, 142–143
    insulin requirements, 144
    monitoring fetal well-being, 143
  effect on maternal diabetes, 145
  fertility in diabetics, 137
  fetal complications, 137, 143
  gestational diabetes, 137, 145
  increased serum TBG, 6
  insulin antagonism, 138–139, 141
  ketoacidosis, 142
  management, 141–143
    diet therapy, 141
    insulin therapy, 141

Index

salt restriction, 141
management of newborn, 144–145
metabolic changes, 138–139
perinatal mortality, 137, 139
risk factors, 140
screening for diabetes, 139–140
Progesterone, diabetes and pregnancy, 138
Propranolol, 15
Propylthiouracil, antithyroid agent, 28
Proteins, lipoprotein composition, 157
Pulmonary function, effect of hypothyroidism, 23
Pyelonephritis, 142–143

Radioimmunoassay methods
serum iodine measurements, 13–14
serum T3 measurements, 14, 39–40
serum TSH concentrations, 2
Radioiodine, thyroidal uptake and suppression tests, 8
Renal calculi
hypercalcinurias
causes of, 98–99
diagnostic criteria for, 99–102
therapy in, 102–106
diphosphonates, 105–106
orthophosphates, 103–105
sodium cellulose phosphate, 102–103
thiazides, 105
medical management of, 97–106
stone formation in, 97–98
Renal function, hypothyroidism and, 23
Renal stones, 97–106
causes of hypercalciuria, 98–99
stone formation, 97–98
Renin
plasma renin activity, 74
and aldosterone, 85
low-renin hypertension, 76–77
Renin-angiotensin-aldosterone system, 73–81
hypertension and hyperaldosteronism, 76
low-renin hypertension, 76–79
physiology of, 73–76
screening procedures, 79–80
Renin-angiotensin system, 49, 74
Respiratory depression, and hypothyroidism, 22, 23
Respiratory distress syndrome, 142

in neonatal period, 143
Retardation, effect of hypothyroidism, 20
Retinal detachment, 148–150
Retinopathy, diabetic, 145, 147–151
incidence of, 147
natural history of, 148
nonproliferative changes in, 148
pathogenesis of, 148
prevention of, 148
proliferative, 148
retinal detachment and, 148–149
treatment of, 148–150
macular edema, 148–149
neovascular glaucoma, 149
photocoagulation treatment, 149
retinal detachment, 149–150
vitrectomy, 150–151
vitreous hemorrhage, 148–150

Salt restriction, 54
Schmidt's syndrome, 50
Serum luteinizing hormone level, 89
Sheehan's syndrome, 4–5, 28
Skin, effect of hypothyroidism on, 20–21
Sodium bicarbonate, diabetic ketoacidosis therapy, 134–135
Sodium cellulose phosphate for hypercalcinurias, 102–103
Sodium loading test, 85
Sodium retention, 54
renin-angiotensin-aldosterone system and, 73–76
Stein-Leventhal syndrome, 89–91
Steroid hormones, 49, 52
diagnosis of Cushing's syndrome, 57
hypertension and, 78
Sulfonylurea drugs, 126–128
contraindications for, 126–127

T3. See Triiodothyronine
T4. See Thyroxine
TBG. See Thyroid binding globulin
Testosterone, 53
serum testosterone test, 89
Thiazides
effect on carbohydrate intolerance, 111

Thiazides, *continued*
  in renal hypercalcinurias, 105
Thyroglobulin, therapy of hypothyroidism, 33
Thyroid binding globulin (TBG), 5
  factors altering concentrations, 6
Thyroid function tests, 1, 32
  clinical appraisal of patient, 7
  diagnosis, 8
  hypothalamic/pituitary interactions, 2–5
  laboratory tests, 7–15
    circulating thyroid hormone levels, 8, 13–15
    hypothalamic/pituitary/thyroid relationship, 8–13
    tissue oxidative metabolism, 8, 15
  to localize anatomic sites of dysfunction, 1
  peripheral tissue actions of thyroid hormones, 7
  physiologic evaluation, 1–17
  thyroid hormone transport in the circulation, 5–7
Thyroid gland
  desiccated, 33
  developmental defects, 27
Thyroid hormones
  biosynthesis and secretion, 1–2, 27–28
  peripheral tissue action, 7
    hypothyroidism and, 29
    laboratory tests, 8, 15
  relationship to biogenic amine metabolism, 7
  secretions, 1–2, 27–28
  tissue metabolism system, 1
  transport in circulation, 1, 5–7
    laboratory tests, 8, 13–15
"Thyroid storm" syndrome, 40
Thyroidectomy, hypothyroidism following, 20, 26–27
Thyroiditis, 4
  atrophic, 25–26
  chronic, 5
  chronic autoimmune, 24, 26
  thyroid enlargement, 26
Thyrotoxic syndromes, 4
  T3 toxicosis, 4
  T4 toxicosis, 4
  T4/T3 thyrotoxicosis, 4
Thyrotoxicosis
  ectopic, 4
  incipient with T3 secretion, 4

  oxygen spirometry to diagnose, 15
  T3, 14
  thyrotropic, 4
Thyrotropin releasing hormone (TRH), 2, 4–5
  provocative tests, 8–9
Thyrotropin stimulation hormone (TSH), 2–3, 19
  increased secretion, 19
  serum concentrations and
    chronic autoimmune thyroiditis, 26, 30
    differential aspects of hypothyroidism, 5, 30
    thyroxine therapy, 33
  serum immunoreactive levels, 8–9
Thyroxine (T4), 3
  deiodination, 7
  laboratory tests, 29
  radioassay procedures, 13
  serum concentration, 29
  serum total T4 and FT4, 13–14
  therapy of hypothyroidism, 33
  thyroid gland secretion into circulation, 5–7
Thyroxine binding prealbumin (TBPA), 5
Tolbutamide, 107, 126
TRH. *See* Thyrotropin releasing hormone
Triglycerides, 154–155
  hypertriglyceridemia, 162–164
  hypothyroidism, 24
  lipoprotein composition, 157
  polyunsaturated, 154
Triiodothyronine (T3), 3
  background, 37–39
  diagnostic value of, 44–45
  discovery of, 37
  euthyroidism with abnormal levels of, 43
  gas-liquid chromatographic methods for measuring, 38–39
  laboratory tests, 29, 38–40
  physiologic and biologic significance, 37–38
  radioimmunoassay procedures for measuring, 37, 39–40
  reverse, 7
  serum total T3 and FT3 concentrations, 14
  sources of, 42
  thyroid hormone transport in circulation, 5–7
  toxicosis, 37–47
Triiodothyronine (T3) toxicosis, 37–47
  clinical variants, 4, 41–42

Index

in course of drug therapy, 41
current role in diagnosis of thyroid disease, 44–45
diagnosis of, 38, 40
discordance between circulating level and clinical state, 42–43
euthyroidism with abnormal levels, 43
hyperthyroidism, 43–44
hypothyroidism, 33, 43
iodine deficiency and, 41–42
after radioactive iodine therapy, 4
reverse, 15
sources in circulation, 42
Tumors
differentiating from bilateral adrenal hyperplasia, 66–68
hypothyroidism and, 5

Urinary 17-hydroxycorticosteroid excretion per gram of creatinine, 57–58
Urinary 17-ketosteroids, differentiating tumors and bilateral adrenal hyperplasia, 66–68
Urine
ketones in, 131
renal stone formation, 97–106

Vitamine B_{12} malabsorption, hypothyroidism, 23, 24
Vitrectomy, treatment of diabetic retinopathy, 150–151

Wolff-Chaikoff effect, 3

Upstate Author